Options for Ensuring Safe Elections

Preparing for Elections During a Pandemic

QUENTIN E. HODGSON, JENNIFER KAVANAGH, ANUSREE GARG, EDWARD W. CHAN, CHRISTINE SOVAK

For more information on this publication, visit www.rand.org/t/RRA112-10

Library of Congress Cataloging-in-Publication Data is available for this publication.
ISBN: 978-1-9774-0555-5

Published by the RAND Corporation, Santa Monica, Calif.
© Copyright 2020 RAND Corporation
RAND® is a registered trademark.

Cover image: Rosemarie/Adobe Stock

Support RAND
Make a tax-deductible charitable contribution at
www.rand.org/giving/contribute

www.rand.org

Preface

In this report, we present and analyze options for voting amid potentially extended threats resulting from the coronavirus disease 2019 (COVID-19) pandemic. We evaluate options based on their abilities to provide a safe means to register and vote, ensure equal access, and protect the integrity of the voting process; we also account for the necessary logistics, costs, timelines, and legislative requirements for implementation. The report is intended to inform policymakers, state and local elected officials, state legislatures, and election officials as they prepare for the 2020 election. The report will also be of interest to other stakeholders, including the voting public.

This report is part of the RAND Corporation's Countering Truth Decay initiative, which is focused on restoring the role of facts, data, and analysis in U.S. political and civil discourse and the policymaking process. The original report, *Truth Decay: An Initial Exploration of the Diminishing Role of Facts and Analysis in American Public Life*, was published in January 2018 and laid out a research agenda for studying and developing solutions to the Truth Decay challenge.[1] Truth Decay worsens when individuals lose trust in institutions that could serve as sources of factual information. Elections that are perceived to be safe, conducted with integrity, and accessible to all eligible voters can be a first step toward building and maintaining a government that people trust. In this report, we examine options for voter registration and

---

[1] Jennifer Kavanagh and Michael D. Rich, *Truth Decay: An Initial Exploration of the Diminishing Role of Facts and Analysis in American Public Life*, Santa Monica, Calif.: RAND Corporation, RR-2314-RC, 2018.

voting and the safety, integrity, access, and logistical implications of each to inform planning for the impact of the pandemic on the 2020 election.

Funding

Funding for RAND's Countering Truth Decay research initiative is provided by gifts from RAND supporters and income from operations. RAND would like to recognize the Joel and Joanne Mogy Truth Decay Fellowship, established by the Mogys in 2020 to support research on Truth Decay, civics, and democracy. The authors drew from the Mogys' generous gift to fund this project.

Contents

Figures and Tables

Figures

Tables

Summary

As the coronavirus disease 2019 (COVID-19) pandemic led governors and local officials to issue stay-at-home orders and the federal government to recommend social distancing, states that had not yet held their primary elections had to scramble to address the pandemic and decide whether to delay their primaries or press ahead.[1] Even as states have begun the process of easing restrictions on businesses and public gatherings, they are warily eyeing autumn for a possible continued spread of COVID-19 and what it might mean for the general election in November.[2]

Scientists, public health officials, and epidemiologists are debating the trajectory of the COVID-19 pandemic, but it appears increasingly likely that there will be a continued need this fall for public health interventions—such as social distancing, limiting the occupancy of close indoor spaces, and aggressive sanitizing protocols—to limit the spread of the disease and protect the public.[3]

---

[1]   Natasha Korecki and Zach Montellaro, "Wisconsin Supreme Court Overturns Governor, Orders Tuesday Elections to Proceed," *Politico*, April 6, 2020.

[2]   Christopher Brito, "CDC Director Says Potentially Worse Second Wave of Coronavirus Could Come Along with Flu Season," CBS News, April 23, 2020. Also see Kristine A. Moore, Marc Lipsitch, John M. Barry, and Michael T. Osterholm, *COVID-19: The CIDRAP Viewpoint,* Part 1, *The Future of the COVID-19 Pandemic: Lessons Learned from Pandemic Influenza*, Minneapolis, Minn.: Center for Infectious Disease Research and Policy, University of Minnesota, April 30, 2020.

[3]   Brito, 2020; Moore et al., 2020. For projections on the pandemic, see Institute for Health Metrics and Evaluation, "COVID-19 Projections," webpage, July 14, 2020. This and similar models provide projections based on current known conditions and assumptions regarding

The question, then, is how the United States can hold its election in November safely and securely under continuing pandemic conditions. Some have recommended that solutions be enacted and applied universally, such as allowing for vote-by-mail in every state.[4] But elections in the United States are administered and run at the state and local levels, which means that state laws govern how elections for federal offices should occur.[5] Each state will have to make decisions in the coming weeks and months about how to conduct the general election in a manner that promotes public health and safety while preserving the integrity of the election.

In this report, we

- outline the options available to states to ensure the safety of elections under pandemic conditions
- provide insights into the factors that election officials, elected officials, policymakers and leaders will have to examine in determining how to conduct the election safely
- weigh the advantages and challenges of each approach and assess the level of risk along several dimensions drawing on past research
- offer insights into how to implement a potential portfolio of options.

The factors we examine are outlined in Table S.1.

---

not only the future course of the virus itself but also public health interventions instituted by various states and localities.

[4]   For example, see Priscilla Southwell, "In the Pandemic, Every State Should Vote by Mail," *The Atlantic*, April 14, 2020; Matt Barreto, Chad Dunn, Vivian Alejandre, Michael Cohen, Tye Rush, and Sonni Waknin, *Protecting Democracy: Implementing Equal and Safe Access to the Ballot Box During a Global Pandemic*, Los Angeles, Calif.: UCLA Latino Policy and Politics Initiative, March 23, 2020; and Lily Hay Newman, "Vote by Mail Isn't Perfect. But It's Essential in a Pandemic," *Wired*, April 9, 2020.

[5]   Michael T. Morley and Franita Tolson, "Elections Clause," *Interactive Constitution* website, undated.

Table S.1
Factors for Analyzing Options for Registration and Voting

Factor	Considerations
Safety	Does the option promote physical safety for the voting public and protect workers from health risks associated with COVID-19?
Integrity	Does the option maintain the integrity of the registration and voting processes, addressing fraud and undue influence and ensuring privacy?
Access	Does the option provide fair and equitable access for all eligible voting populations without undue burden?
Logistics	What steps are needed to implement the option in terms of planning, timelines, costs, and materials?

Assessment of Factors for Voter Registration Options

Table S.2 summarizes the considerations across the four factors for the most-prevalent forms of voter registration: in-person, online, and mail-in. We do not factor in considerations that apply equally to all options—for example, all options must provide accommodations for non-English speakers and voters with disabilities. The most useful way

Table S.2
Summary of Risks for Implementing Voter Registration Options During a Pandemic

	Risks to Safety	Risks to Integrity	Risks to Access	Logistical Considerations
In-person	High • New interpersonal contact • Automatic voter registration (AVR) could reduce risk	Minimal	Moderate • Travel required	Safety and sanitation mitigations • Communication • Training
Online	Minimal	Low (but higher than in-person) • Cybersecurity	Low • Internet availability • Technology requirements	Online system, processing • Verification • Training • Communication
Mail-in	Minimal	Low (but higher than in-person)	Minimal	Processing and verification • Training • Verification

to consider these assessments is in relative terms. The table indicates that risks associated with safety (specifically that associated with physical health related to COVID-19) are highest for in-person registration. Inferring from past research, risks associated with access are highest for in-person registration (because of the need to travel to an outside location), somewhat lower for online registration, and lowest for mail-in registration.[6] However, it is also worth noting that AVR, which can occur in person, might increase access and reduce this risk by conducting registration as part of another registration process (albeit in person).[7] Risks associated with integrity are low across the board but likely to be slightly higher for remote options, as is the case with voting.[8] However, all options have significant logistical considerations. For in-person registration, logistical considerations focus on safety. For online and mail-in options, the logistical considerations are largely focused on creating systems (if they are not already in place) to support remote processes and acquiring the equipment needed for processing submitted registrations. It is difficult to rank the logistical challenges associated with different voting systems by size or severity.

Considering across options and assessing each factor equally, risk seems relatively lower for online and mail-in options compared with in-person options, at least in the pandemic context we focus on here. However, different states might weight these four factors differently. For some, integrity might be the priority, for others access, for others safety. Ultimately, the options chosen by a given state will reflect the

---

[6]   Jeffrey A. Karp and Susan A. Banducci, "Going Postal: How All-Mail Elections Influence Turnout," *Political Behavior*, Vol. 22, No. 3, 2000; Priscilla L. Southwell and Justin I. Burchett, "The Effect of All-Mail Elections on Voter Turnout," *American Politics Quarterly*, Vol. 28, No. 1, 2000.

[7]   Daniel P. Franklin and Eric E. Grier, "Effects of Motor Voter Legislation: Voter Turnout, Registration, and Partisan Advantage in the 1992 Presidential Election," *American Politics Quarterly*, Vol. 25, No. 1, 1997; Stephen Knack, "Does 'Motor Voter' Work? Evidence from State-Level Data," *Journal of Politics*, Vol. 57, No. 3, 1995.

[8]   Robert M. Stein, *The Incidence and Detection of Ineligible Voting*, paper presented at American Political Science Association 2013 annual meeting, 2013; Sharad Goel, Marc Meredith, Michael Morse, David Rothschild, and Houshmand Shirani-Mehr, "One Person, One Vote: Estimating the Prevalence of Double Voting in U.S. Presidential Elections," *American Political Science Review*, Vol. 114, No. 2, May 2020.

priorities of state policymakers and election officials and the constraints of existing policies and laws.

Assessment of Factors for Voting Options

Table S.3 outlines the options available for voting and discusses the relevant considerations for each of these dimensions, again drawing on relevant academic research. As already noted, we do not factor in considerations that apply equally to all options—for example, all options must provide accommodations for non-English speakers and voters with disabilities. Safety risks are highest for in-person voting, at least in the COVID-19 context. Mitigations are available to help reduce this risk but will involve additional effort and cost. The safety considerations associated with voting on Election Day and voting early are

Table S.3
Summary of Risks for Implementing Voting Options During a Pandemic

	Risks to Safety	Risks to Integrity	Risks to Access	Logistical Considerations
In-person (Election Day or early voting)	High (potentially lower with early voting) • New interpersonal contact	Minimal • Possible identification requirement	Moderate • Travel required • Possible identification requirement • Physical requirement	Safety and sanitation mitigations • Communication • Physical space or modifications • Training
Mail (absentee or mail-in)	Minimal	Low (but higher than in-person) • Increased volume of mail-in ballots might increase risk (e.g., harder to detect fraud)	Minimal	Dissemination • Processing and verification • Training • Verification
Other (online or fax)	Minimal	High • Cybersecurity • Technical failures	Low • Internet availability • Technology requirements	Online system, processing • Verification • Training • Communication

similar; both are in-person processes, although early voting can help spread voters out and reduce the challenges associated with social distancing. Past research indicates that access considerations appear lowest for mail-in voting because eligible voters can do this from home with less investment of time in most cases, although even this approach can create hurdles for some voters. Access concerns are somewhat higher for in-person voting methods (which require people to travel to the polls) and for online voting options,[9] which require access to specific technology and to reliable internet connectivity.[10] Early voting also could have some positive effect on increasing access if it offers more flexibility to voters and allows them to vote more easily. However, it is worth noting that research finds only muted effects of early voting on turnout.[11] Integrity concerns are lowest for in-person voting methods and highest for online approaches. Although the risk of fraud is potentially higher for mail-in options than for in-person voting, this risk can remain very low overall if proper safeguards, such as signature verification, are implemented.[12] Finally, as is true for registration, there are significant pandemic-related logistical considerations across options. It is hard to compare these options based on scale or to assess which set of logistical considerations is most or least severe. Instead, we assess that, regardless of the options chosen, local officials will need to address a variety of logistical issues, whether these result from physical safety

---

[9] Online voting is available only to voters eligible under the Uniformed and Overseas Citizens Absentee Voting Act (UOCAVA) and, in some states, to voters in a few defined classes, such as those with disabilities, but we consider the option here anyway.

[10] Jennifer Stromer-Galley, "Will Internet Voting Increase Turnout?" in Philip N. Howard and Steve Jones, eds., *Society Online: The Internet in Context*, Washington, D.C.: SAGE Publications, 2003, p. 87; Mihkel Solvak and Kristjan Vassil, "Could Internet Voting Halt Declining Electoral Turnout? New Evidence That E-Voting Is Habit-Forming," *Policy & Internet*, Vol. 10, No. 1, 2018; Karp and Banducci, 2000; Southwell and Burchett, 2000.

[11] Paul Gronke, Eva Galanes-Rosenbaum, and Peter A. Miller, "Early Voting and Turnout," *PS: Political Science & Politics*, Vol. 40, No. 4, 2007; Robert M. Stein, "Introduction: Early Voting," *Public Opinion Quarterly*, Vol. 62, No. 1, 1998.

[12] Commission on Federal Election Reform, *Building Confidence in U.S. Elections: Report of The Commission on Federal Election Reform*, September 2005; Reality Check Team, "US Election: Do Postal Ballots Lead to Voting Fraud?" BBC, July 15, 2020; Jason Snead, *The Unnecessary Risks of Mandated and Rushed Vote-by-Mail*, Honest Elections Project, 2020.

and sanitation issues or from the technical requirements of disseminating, collecting, and processing mail-in ballots. The most-significant logistical considerations are listed in the table, which is intended not to be exhaustive but to highlight some of the most-significant pandemic-relevant logistical concerns.

We can also compare across options, looking specifically at which voting options present the most risks and considerations for local officials within the pandemic context. Table S.3 would seem to indicate that local officials face more mitigation requirements and more considerations about logistics and safety regarding in-person elections than for mail-in voting. Once again, however, this assessment is particular to the current context and might look different in non-pandemic times. Furthermore, the risks and considerations across options might have different relevance and different implications in different states. Ultimately, each state must weigh the considerations outlined here and decide which mix of approaches is best. Some states might lean toward mail-in voting options that have less safety risk. For others, in-person options might be preferred because of logistical considerations or integrity concerns. Notably, states will be constrained in their choices by political and legal considerations and by the time remaining before the election to implement any changes. State and local level officials, supported by their federal government partners, will also have to remain vigilant in the face of potential foreign interference, whether through disinformation campaigns or cyber threats to election infrastructure, in the election.

Given that each option carries risk in different areas, election officials likely will have to consider a portfolio approach that balances the risks that they are willing to assume. To assist with determining a risk-informed path forward, we offer the following set of filtering questions for state officials to ask themselves:

What is our starting point in terms of election systems and voter preferences? States where most people have historically voted in person are at a different starting point than states where universal vote-by-mail has been implemented, particularly when viewed from a perspective of safety. Similar considerations apply to registration methods.

What types of risks are we willing to accept? What are our risk priorities? States vary in the extent to which they feel that changes to their election processes are required or desirable. Although all states might choose to implement some health-related precautions at in-person voting locations, some states might lean toward efforts to expand mail-in voting while others might prefer to continue with existing processes augmented by additional polling locations or expanded early voting. Although many factors will be considered, at least part of the decision will be based on the preferences and risk tolerance of key stakeholders, such as policymakers and elections officials.

How much flexibility is there to make changes to our existing approach? States also have different laws and regulations around voting and vary in the ease with which they can modify policy and practice on the timeline required. States and jurisdictions that have less flexibility, such as those that require legislative changes to allow for absentee ballots that do not require an excuse or vote-by-mail could have fewer choices in the near term when it comes to changing voting methods and might instead choose to focus more closely on implementing safety precautions and communicating those measures broadly to the voting public.[13]

Given estimates of uncertainty and voter preferences, do we have the capacity to meet voter demands for different types of voting options? Historical experience and estimates of 2020 turnout and voter preferences (which could be gleaned from new or existing studies) indicate that state officials should be able to produce rough estimates of how many eligible voters might turn out to vote in person on Election Day, vote early, or take advantage of mail-in options (where those exist). Such estimates could allow state officials to determine whether existing capacity is sufficient for in-person, mail-in, and other options—and if it is not, what additional mix of policy options might be required to meet demand (for example, more in-person locations or additional in-person mitigations and some additional remote

---

[13] Our companion report provides more detail on which states have greater or less flexibility as determined by their laws and systems. See Jennifer Kavanagh, Quentin E. Hodgson, C. Ben Gibson, and Samantha Cherney, *An Assessment of State Voting Processes: Preparing for Elections During a Pandemic*, Santa Monica, Calif.: RAND Corporation, RR-A112-8, 2020.

voting capacity) and what additional costs (both monetary and potentially political) these modifications might entail. Finally, it is worth noting that to truly hedge against uncertainty, planners might choose to slightly overestimate demand across methods or develop the capacity to rapidly shift staff or resources from one voting method to another as late as Election Day; if they do so, these changes should be broadly communicated to the voting public.

Elected officials, policymakers, and election officials face extraordinary circumstances preparing for the November election. Planning for such uncertain conditions will require careful evaluation and likely additional funding from states—and the federal government, given the strain on state and local budgets stemming from the response to the pandemic.

Acknowledgments

The authors thank the donors to RAND for their generous support, without which this work would not be possible. We thank our reviewers—Geoff McGovern, Michael Pollard, Juliette Kayyem, Brian Jenkins, Christopher Deluzio, Scott Bates, and Jim Thomson—for their careful and insightful reviews and comments. We also thank Henry Willis, Jordan Fischbach, Erica Robles, and Steph Bingley for shepherding this report through review and publication. The authors are grateful for the assistance of Arwen Bicknell, who edited the report. Finally, but no less importantly, we thank Michael Rich for his strong support.

Abbreviations

AVR	automatic voter registration
COVID-19	coronavirus disease 2019
DMV	Department of Motor Vehicles
PPE	personal protective equipment
UOCAVA	Uniformed and Overseas Citizens Absentee Voting Act

CHAPTER ONE

Introduction

The coronavirus disease 2019 (COVID-19) pandemic sweeping the nation has caused massive social and economic upheaval. During much of the spring, cities fell quiet, streets emptied, and many businesses shuttered their doors—many of which might never open again. 2020 is also a presidential election year in the United States, which normally would mean large rallies, fundraising dinners, and candidates of all stripes up and down the ballot engaging with the American people in a bid to secure their votes. More than half of the states held their primary elections prior to the enactment of stay-at-home orders and social distancing advisories that began in March 2020, but the remainder had to decide whether to delay their primaries or press ahead—often scrambling to implement new procedures, address a sudden shortage of pollworkers, and address legal challenges to proposed mitigations.[1] Twelve states,[2] the U.S. Virgin Islands, and Puerto Rico all delayed their presidential primary elections; elsewhere, voters were encouraged to take advantage of early voting, absentee voting, or vote-by-mail. Even as states have begun the process of easing restrictions on businesses and public gatherings, they are warily eyeing autumn for the continued

---

[1] Natasha Korecki and Zach Montellaro, "Wisconsin Supreme Court Overturns Governor, Orders Tuesday Elections to Proceed," *Politico*, April 6, 2020.

[2] Those states were Connecticut, Delaware, Georgia, Indiana, Kentucky, Louisiana, Maryland, New Jersey, New York, Pennsylvania, Rhode Island, and West Virginia. Some states and territories have postponed multiple times: Connecticut, Georgia, Guam, Louisiana, New Jersey, and Puerto Rico.

spread of the pandemic and what it might mean for the general election in November.[3]

It is possible, even likely, that there will be a continued need for public health interventions through 2020, and possibly beyond—such as social distancing, limiting occupancy of close indoor spaces, and aggressive sanitizing protocols.[4] Although many states responded to the public health threat by postponing primary elections by several months in hopes that the situation would improve, Congress has little flexibility for moving the November elections. The date for choosing the electors for the President of the United States was established in law by the 28th Congress in 1845, which stated that the electors should be selected on the first Tuesday after the first Monday in November of an election year.[5] The 20th Amendment moved the date for inaugurating the president from March 4 to January 20 in the year following the election. Therefore, although the Constitution grants Congress the authority to potentially change the date of the general election, there is only so far the date could move without affecting the convening of the electoral college and the constitutionally required inauguration date.

How can the United States hold its election in November safely, ensure access for eligible voters, and protect the integrity of the voting process under potential continuing pandemic conditions? Elections in the United States are administered and run at the state and local

---

[3]   Christopher Brito, "CDC Director Says Potentially Worse Second Wave of Coronavirus Could Come Along with Flu Season," CBS News, April 23, 2020. Also see Kristine A. Moore, Marc Lipsitch, John M. Barry, and Michael T. Osterholm, *COVID-19: The CIDRAP Viewpoint,* Part 1, *The Future of the COVID-19 Pandemic: Lessons Learned from Pandemic Influenza,* Minneapolis, Minn.: Center for Infectious Disease Research and Policy, University of Minnesota, April 30, 2020; and Stephen M. Kissler, Christine Tedijanto, Edward Goldstein, Yonatan H. Grad, and Marc Lipsitch, "Projecting the Transmission Dynamics of SARS-CoV-2 Through the Postpandemic Period," *Science,* Vol. 368, No. 6493, 2020.

[4]   It is challenging to predict with high confidence the future course of the response to the COVID-19 pandemic because of several factors—such as possible seasonal variations in transmission; how long previously infected people maintain immunity; and the intensity, timing, and duration of control measures implemented. See Kissler et al., 2020. For projections on the pandemic, see Institute for Health Metrics and Evaluation, "COVID-19 Projections," webpage, July 14, 2020.

[5]   3 U.S. Code § 1, Time of Appointing Electors.

levels, which means that state laws govern how elections for federal offices should occur.[6] Each state has a different approach to how it conducts elections, influenced by experience over many years and the relative weight of authority allocated between state and local jurisdictions in implementing and running elections. (Our companion report provides an in-depth examination of how each state conducts registration and voting.[7]) Despite the different approaches, some have recommended that solutions be enacted and applied universally, such as allowing for vote-by-mail in every state.[8] Oregon has the longest experience with running elections by mail, and four other states have joined it in implementing this approach (Colorado; Washington; Utah; and, most recently, Hawaii). Other states have lower rates of participation by absentee ballot—in some cases, this is because a valid excuse is required to request a ballot (hereafter referred to as *excuse-required*); in others, it stems from a lack of a concerted push to promote voting outside the polling place.[9] Each state, then, will have to make decisions in the coming weeks and months about how it will seek to conduct the general election in a manner that promotes public health and safety while preserving access for eligible voters and the integrity of the election. State and local level officials, supported by their federal government partners, will also have to remain vigilant in the face of potential foreign interference, whether through disinformation campaigns or cyber threats to election infrastructure, in the election. A one-size-

---

[6]   Michael T. Morley and Franita Tolson, "Elections Clause," *Interactive Constitution* website, undated.

[7]   Jennifer Kavanagh, Quentin E. Hodgson, C. Ben Gibson, and Samantha Cherney, *An Assessment of State Voting Processes: Preparing for Elections During a Pandemic*, Santa Monica, Calif.: RAND Corporation, RR-A112-8, 2020.

[8]   For example, see Amy Klobuchar, "Amy Klobuchar: The Right Way to Vote This November," *New York Times*, April 14, 2020; Priscilla Southwell, "In the Pandemic, Every State Should Vote by Mail," *The Atlantic*, April 14, 2020; Matt Barreto, Chad Dunn, Vivian Alejandre, Michael Cohen, Tye Rush, and Sonni Waknin, *Protecting Democracy: Implementing Equal and Safe Access to the Ballot Box During a Global Pandemic*, Los Angeles, Calif.: UCLA Latino Policy and Politics Initiative, March 23, 2020; and Lily Hay Newman, "Vote by Mail Isn't Perfect. But It's Essential in a Pandemic," *Wired*, April 9, 2020.

[9]   Nathaniel Rakich, "Few States Are Prepared to Switch to Voting by Mail. That Could Make for a Messy Election," *FiveThirtyEight*, April 27, 2020.

fits-all approach is unlikely to work, but time to plan and prepare for the November election is running out, and uncertainty remains high regarding which options make the most sense, so states will need to work quickly to assess their own preparedness and to implement contingency plans where needed.

In this report, we

- outline options that are available to states to ensure the safety, integrity, and accessibility of elections under pandemic conditions
- provide insights into the factors election officials and leaders will have to examine
- weigh the advantages and challenges of each approach and assess the level of risk along several dimensions, drawing on past research
- offer insights into how to implement a potential portfolio of options.

This analysis is intended to inform election officials, policymakers, and elected officials at the federal, state, and local levels, as well as the voting public. This is so that voters and public officials alike have the greatest possible confidence that they can participate in and conduct elections safely, supporting access for eligible voters and maintaining the integrity of the voting process. In the next chapter, we provide an overview of options for voter registration and for casting ballots, followed by a discussion of the factors we use to evaluate each option. We then bring the two together to evaluate the options and discuss implementation considerations.

CHAPTER TWO

How the United States Votes

The elections process is a series of steps that precede Election Day and extend through the certification of results and beyond. There are discrete events, such as vote tabulation, and ongoing processes, such as registration. In presidential election years, we can expect significant efforts on the parts of both major political parties to motivate supporters and improve their chances at the polls, including efforts to register new voters and promote turnout. In this chapter, we focus on the process of registering and voting, from the point of registration through the submission and processing of the ballot.

Figure 2.1 gives an overview of available options that state and local policymakers and officials can consider as they establish election procedures. In the material that follows, we describe the options and discuss a set of considerations that policymakers should consider when making choices across options and when investing in specific processes or technologies.

Options for Voter Registration

Although states vary in their types of registration processes and systems, all states (except North Dakota) have to maintain voter registration databases that reflect new voter registrations, update existing registrations, and remove obsolete records (for example, voters who have moved out of

Figure 2.1
Overview of Registration and Voting Options

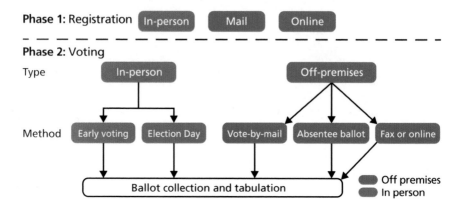

state or jurisdiction or have died).[1] Thirty-nine states are so-called *top-down* states, where the voter registration database of record is operated at the state level. Local jurisdictions take voter registration information and feed it to the state level. Other *bottom-up* states rely on local jurisdictions to maintain registration databases at the local level, and the state maintains the aggregated data. A few states, such as Texas, employ a hybrid system in which the state maintains the voter registration database for most jurisdictions but some maintain their own.

Prospective voters can register to vote in several ways:

- with the local elections office, such as a county clerk or registrar; options to do so also might be available online or by mail
- at the Department of Motor Vehicles (DMV)
- at other state agencies that provide public assistance
- through a third-party voter registration organization, such as a registration drive.[2]

---

[1]   The 2002 Help America Vote Act requires that states maintain a statewide voter registration database. North Dakota is the one exception because it allows state residents to appear on Election Day and vote with valid identification. See National Conference of State Legislatures, "Voter List Accuracy," webpage, March 20, 2020c; and National Conference of State Legislatures, "Voter Registration," webpage, September 27, 2016.

[2]   National Conference of State Legislatures, 2016.

Online voter registration mirrors paper-based processes in seeking similar information from the prospective voter but can reduce errors because the application is submitted electronically and does not require transferring the information from paper to create a computer record.[3] Thirty-nine states and the District of Columbia have online voter registration.[4] Oklahoma allows registered voters to make online updates to their registration records (for example, change of address) but has not yet implemented full online registration.[5] Once a prospective voter submits an application, it has to be verified by election officials. Normally, this consists of validating that the given home address is a legitimate address; it could require some form of validation of documentation, such as matching driver's license numbers to DMV records or verifying a Social Security number against the Social Security Administration's database. Fourteen states and the District of Columbia have adopted automatic voter registration (AVR) systems that automatically register eligible voters or update information during interactions with certain state agencies. Therefore, AVR can improve the accuracy of voter registration rolls.[6]

Options for Receiving and Casting a Ballot

For the majority of U.S. voters, there are three main options for voting in an election: in person, by absentee ballot, or by mail. *Voting in person* refers to early voting or voting on Election Day at voting centers, polling places, or the registrar's office. Polling places need to check in voters using a pollbook and provide them with the means to vote via a paper ballot to be hand-marked and scanned or via a computer-

---

[3] It does rely on the voter entering their own information correctly.

[4] National Conference of State Legislatures, "Online Voter Registration," webpage, February 3, 2020b.

[5] The status of Oklahoma's system is from Oklahoma State Election Board, "Online Voter Registration," webpage, November 1, 2019.

[6] Eric McGhee and Mindy Romero, *Effects of Automatic Voter Registration in the United States*, Los Angeles, Calif.: USC Sol Price School of Public Policy, 2020, p. 4.

ized machine (that is, a ballot-marking device or a direct recording electronic machine) that will record a voter's choices (with or without a paper record, depending on the system). The process for voting in person also has to provide assistance to voters who need accommodations for disabilities or who cannot physically come into the polling center.

Voting with an absentee ballot or vote-by-mail are distinct options but have similar considerations in terms of processing. *Absentee ballots* have to be requested by the voter online (if that option is available), through the mail, or by phone. In the context of the COVID-19 pandemic, some states have made exceptions. For example, Michigan and Ohio sent voters a request form automatically for their 2020 primary elections. However, absentee voting still requires a voter to send the request back in time to receive a ballot, which proved challenging in some jurisdictions.[7] Absentee voting also requires that the voter return the ballot by the stated deadline, which can mean it has to be either postmarked or received in the elections office by a certain date (such as on Election Day). This requirement varies by state. Postal service delays and whether postage costs are borne by the jurisdiction or the voter are also important elements to consider.[8]

Vote-by-mail removes the ballot request step in absentee balloting. For states with universal vote-by-mail, election officials mail ballots to registered voters in advance of the election period. Other states have a permanent mail-in ballot option for those who request it, which functions similarly. Ballots are then returned either by mail (with the same type of time requirements as absentee ballots) or to ballot drop-boxes at polling places or registrars' offices. Most states have some form of verification process, such as a signature verification or a notarized or

---

[7] For example, see Nick Corasaniti and Stephanie Saul, "Requests for Vote-by-Mail Ballot Overwhelm the Elections Agency in New York City," *New York Times*, June 20, 2020.

[8] Of note, most return envelopes will state that postage is required, but the U.S. Postal Service in prior elections has adopted a policy to complete delivery of ballots regardless of postage. See Susie Armitage, "Mail-In Ballot Postage Becomes a Surprising (and Unnecessary) Cause of Voter Anxiety," *ProPublica*, November 1, 2018.

witnessed ballot envelope.[9] For clarity and simplicity in this report, we address absentee ballots and vote-by-mail together, but we do discuss where the factors for each form of voting differ.

Congress enacted the Uniformed and Overseas Citizens Absentee Voting Act (UOCAVA) in 1986 to ensure that deployed members of the military, their families, and other U.S. citizens living overseas could vote in elections. The program is administered by the U.S. Department of Defense's Federal Voting Assistance Program.[10] UOCAVA voters can receive a blank ballot via fax or email and return the completed ballot through the mail (or sometimes by fax or email, depending on state regulations).[11]

Voting electronically through email or online through a web portal is not an option for most voters except for those covered by UOCAVA and in a few instances in which states and local jurisdictions have experimented with online voting.[12] Utah, for example, allows voters with disabilities to return their ballots via email or fax.[13]

---

[9] For a detailed description of the types of verification and states requiring them, see Kavanagh et al., 2020.

[10] Federal Voting Assistance Program, homepage, undated-b.

[11] Federal Voting Assistance Program, "Election Forms and Tools for Sending," webpage, undated-a.

[12] Mia Logan, "These States Allow Online Voting for Citizens, Is Your State One of Them?" *eBallot* blog, May 16, 2019.

[13] State of Utah, "Information for Voters with Disabilities," webpage, undated.

CHAPTER THREE

Factors to Consider in Preparing Election Systems for Response to the Pandemic

In the previous chapter, we outlined the options that states have when considering how best to execute elections. In making those choices, states will need to consider several different factors. In this chapter, we discuss each factor that our team used in evaluating the options and how each factor applies both generally and specifically to a pandemic scenario. We also describe how we applied each factor across the different voting options described in the previous chapter. Table 3.1 summarizes the factors.

Safety

As states and local governments seek to implement phased plans for lifting social restrictions, public safety and health are primary concerns and

Table 3.1
Factors for Analyzing Options for Registration and Voting

Factor	Considerations
Safety	Does the option promote physical safety for the voting public and protect workers from health risks associated with COVID-19?
Integrity	Does the option maintain the integrity of the registration and voting processes, addressing fraud and undue influence and ensuring privacy?
Access	Does the option provide fair and equitable access for all eligible voting populations without undue burden?
Logistics	What steps are needed to implement the option in terms of planning, timelines, costs and materials?

will likely remain so into the fall as the general election approaches.[1] Election officials have to ensure not only their own safety but also the safety of the voting public and election workers and/or volunteers; officials also have to communicate the approaches being taken and promote public confidence that the voting process will not pose a risk to physical health. This is particularly important when addressing safety measures for those at higher risk of death or severe complications from COVID-19. People over the age of 65, for example, represent about a quarter of voter turnout while also falling in a higher risk category.[2] In the context of the COVID-19 pandemic, safety is promoted by several specific measures. First, any voting option that promotes social distancing or facilitates remote processes promotes safety. For example, early voting can support safety by providing more days for voters to go to the polls, supporting social distancing by spreading voters over time. Similarly, mail-in options for voting and registration increase safety by reducing person-to-person contact. Sanitation at polling locations and provisions of personal protective equipment (PPE), such as masks and gloves, can also increase safety when they are added to in-person voting processes.

Integrity

Election officials have to maintain the integrity of the registration and voting process to ensure that only legitimate voters are registered and cast ballots, that voters are not subject to undue influence or coercion, and that voter choices are kept confidential. Documented cases of voter fraud are rare, but the potential for fraud varies across different forms of voting.[3] Specifically, research suggests that remote processes, such as mail-in voting, do have a slightly higher rate of fraud than in-

---

[1]   Lena H. Sun, "CDC Director Warns Second Wave of Coronavirus Is Likely to Be Even More Devastating," *Washington Post*, April 21, 2020.

[2]   On voter turnout rates, see Pew Research Center, "An Examination of the 2016 Electorate, Based on Validated Voters," webpage, August 9, 2018.

[3]   Elise Viesbeck, "Tiny Rate of Fraudulent Ballots Undercuts Claims of Risk," *Washington Post*, June 9, 2020.

person options.[4] However, it is essential to emphasize that this rate of fraud remains minuscule across options when compared with the volume of overall voter registrations and votes cast.[5] Furthermore, when surveying a broader set of election processes and policies, research shows that making voting and registration easier for eligible voters has not resulted in increased incidence of fraud. What evidence of fraud has been uncovered and proven tends to be small in scale, often driven by misunderstandings and errors—although fraud does occur. Furthermore, provisions already in place, such as signature matching, appear to be sufficient to maintain the integrity of the mail-in process.[6] There is no evidence to support claims of large-scale fraud perpetrated either by domestic or foreign actors.

When we consider voting options in the remainder of this paper, therefore, we consider the risk of fraud to be lowest for in-person options and only very slightly higher for remote processes, such as mail-in voting. Online processes, however, might be less secure because they face not only traditional threats, such as impersonation, but also cybersecurity vulnerabilities that an adversary could exploit to manipulate elections on larger scale.[7] Implementing a secure online voting system in the remaining months before the November election would be extremely challenging.

Related to integrity is the question of how effectively different modes of voting can be audited after the election in cases where the outcome might be challenged. On this issue, the differences fall less across

---

[4]   Robert M. Stein, *The Incidence and Detection of Ineligible Voting*, paper presented at the American Political Science Association 2013 annual meeting, 2013; Sharad Goel, Marc Meredith, Michael Morse, David Rothschild, and Houshmand Shirani-Mehr, "One Person, One Vote: Estimating the Prevalence of Double Voting in U.S. Presidential Elections," *American Political Science Review*, Vol. 114, No. 2, May 2020.

[5]   This finding has been confirmed by multiple analyses. See Lori Minnite and David Callahan, *Securing the Vote*, New York: Demos, 2003; and Reality Check Team, "US Election: Do Postal Ballots Lead to Voting Fraud?" BBC, July 15, 2020.

[6]   Goel et al., 2020; Minnite and Callahan, 2003; Stein, 2013.

[7]   Kim Zetter, "U.S. Government Plans to Urge States to Resist 'High-Risk' Internet Voting," *The Guardian*, May 8, 2020; Miles Parks, "Feds Warn States That Online Voting Experiments Are 'High-Risk,'" National Public Radio, May 11, 2020b.

modes of voting than types of ballots and the type of audit.[8] Although there are systems that allow for audits of electronic voting, auditing is generally easier for paper ballots that can be reviewed and recounted. Because mail-in ballots are paper ballots, mail-in voting processes might have advantages on this dimension.[9] Of course, paper audits will be affected by human error, so no system is entirely free of risk.

Access

Every citizen of the United States who has attained the age of 18 has the right to vote unless that right has been suspended or revoked (for example, for felony convictions). Election officials seek to ensure that every eligible voter has access to register to vote and cast their ballot without an undue burden, such as for those who have disabilities needing special accommodation, those for whom English is not their primary language, the elderly, and minorities. Different voting options have been shown to have different implications for access, as measured by voter turnout. For example, processes that reduce barriers or increase options for voters (such as remote voting, AVR, and early voting) do appear to increase turnout, although by different amounts across options and less than sometimes assumed.

On early voting, most research suggests a generally small positive effect on aggregate turnout.[10] The effect for mail-in voting appears more sizable. However, in both cases, increases in turnout are largest among those who are already inclined to vote rather than among those who

---

[8]   Post-election audits consist of a recount of some set percentage of ballots cast or a "risk-limiting" audit that uses a statistical sampling of ballots. Additionally, vote tabulation and vote casting equipment can be audited to check that they produce the same results each time given the same inputs.

[9]   Lawrence Norden, Aaron Burstein, Joseph Lorenzo Hall, and Margaret Chen, *Post-Election Audits: Restoring Trust in Elections: Executive Summary*, New York: Brennan Center for Justice and Samuelson Law, Technology & Public Policy Clinic, 2007.

[10]   Paul Gronke, Eva Galanes-Rosenbaum, and Peter A. Miller, "Early Voting and Turnout," *PS: Political Science & Politics*, Vol. 40, No. 4, 2007; Robert M. Stein, "Introduction: Early Voting," *Public Opinion Quarterly*, Vol. 62, No. 1, 1998.

would not have voted without the additional flexibility. The effects of mail-in voting on turnout have also been found to be smaller for presidential elections and other elections with significant consequences.[11]

Although the United States does not have an online voting system for most voters, pilot studies and research from foreign democracies suggests that online voting can have a positive effect on voter turnout, but this effect is more muted than might be expected. Once again, it seems that the greatest shift to this new method of voting is among people who would have voted anyway, not from an influx of new voters.[12] Online voting also has additional access considerations, such as the availability of reliable internet connectivity and necessary technologies (for example, printers and scanners), and the need to ensure that the voting interface functions and displays properly on multiple platforms, operating systems, and web browsers. These barriers might be most likely to constrain the access of poorer and rural voters; research on voting identification laws confirms that such laws do reduce access and turnout, especially for minority groups, although aggregate effects are more modest.[13]

There is limited research on whether different types of registration (for example, in-person, online, or vote-by-mail) significantly affect the number of people who end up registering, but what evidence

---

[11] Jeffrey A. Karp and Susan A. Banducci, "Going Postal: How All-Mail Elections Influence Turnout," *Political Behavior*, Vol. 22, No. 3, 2000; Priscilla L. Southwell and Justin I. Burchett, "The Effect of All-Mail Elections on Voter Turnout," *American Politics Quarterly*, Vol. 28, No. 1, 2000.

[12] Jennifer Stromer-Galley, "Will Internet Voting Increase Turnout?" in Philip N. Howard and Steve Jones, eds., *Society Online: The Internet in Context*, Washington, D.C.: SAGE Publications, 2003, p. 87; Mihkel Solvak and Kristjan Vassil, "Could Internet Voting Halt Declining Electoral Turnout? New Evidence That E-Voting Is Habit-Forming," *Policy & Internet*, Vol. 10, No. 1, 2018.

[13] Zoltan Hajnal, Nazita Lajevardi, and Lindsay Nielson, "Voter Identification Laws and the Suppression of Minority Votes," *Journal of Politics*, Vol. 79, No. 2, 2017; Benjamin Highton, "Voter Identification Laws and Turnout in the United States," *Annual Review of Political Science*, Vol. 20, 2017, pp. 149–167. For an analysis that argues that other factors (such as political issues and socioeconomic factors) have a greater impact than voter identification requirements, see Jason D. Mycoff, Michael W. Wagner, and David C. Wilson, "The Empirical Effects of Voter-ID Laws: Present or Absent?" *Political Science and Politics*, Vol. 41, No. 1, January 2009.

does exist allows us to infer that the effects are likely to be similar to those associated with different forms of voting. We use this research to assess the access implications of voting options. Research does suggest that AVR is associated with increased turnout, although the size of any such relationship is less clear.[14]

When assessing the access implications of different voting options, we consider such options as remote voting, mail-in registration, and AVR to increase access compared with alternatives. We consider online options to have mixed effects because they can reduce barriers for some but create new hurdles for others. Identification requirements are considered to have a negative effect on access.

Notably, there is tension between considerations of access and of integrity. For example, voter identification requirements are sometimes used to ensure election integrity, but critics argue that such requirements pose barriers for some voters. Research on this topic is mixed, but voter identification requirements generally have minimal effect on turnout overall, although there is some evidence that these effects are heaviest on minority voters.[15] Similarly, signature matching processes are used to maintain integrity, but research has indicated that such processes can adversely affect such groups as the young and some minorities, leading to higher rejection rates than for the electorate as a whole.[16]

Logistics

Implementing any option requires careful planning and execution to ensure that the materials, people, and processes are in place to support the option. Normally, changes to voting systems are a steady evolutionary process built on historical experience, and adjustments can be incre-

---

[14] Daniel P. Franklin and Eric E. Grier, "Effects of Motor Voter Legislation: Voter Turnout, Registration, and Partisan Advantage in the 1992 Presidential Election," *American Politics Quarterly*, Vol. 25, No. 1, 1997; Stephen Knack, "Does 'Motor Voter' Work? Evidence from State-Level Data," *Journal of Politics*, Vol. 57, No. 3, 1995.

[15] Highton, 2017; Hajnal, Lajevardi, and Nielson, 2017.

[16] Daniel A. Smith, "Vote-by-Mail Ballots Cast in Florida," ACLU Florida webpage, September 19, 2018.

mental over time.[17] Transitioning to a new approach or greatly increasing registration and voting options carries logistical considerations for which election officials must account, such as planning out timelines to implement processes and secure additional needed funds, which might be considerable.[18] The U.S. Department of Homeland Security's Cybersecurity and Infrastructure Security Agency has issued a series of papers that provides detailed advice on the logistics of vote-by-mail, absentee balloting, and ballot drop-boxes, among other topics.[19] Other issues that are part of this factor are processes for sanitizing and for ensuring social distancing at in-person voting locations and, for some states, the time required to update necessary policies or laws. Finally, communicating any changes and the options available is critical to ensuring that the voting public knows how and where to register and to vote.

For each option, we also provide cost categories to consider. These are not intended to be exhaustive but to identify the major cost drivers and significant logistical challenges that emerge specifically from the pandemic context. More-detailed planning and an assessment of a state's or jurisdiction's circumstances will be necessary to illuminate costs in detail. The logistical demands of each voting option will vary, and it will be challenging to compare across options. For example, in-person voting will require sanitation and provisions for social distancing. It will require PPE for pollworkers, and might call for additional medical and security personnel to enforce guidelines and deal with emergencies. A shift to mail-in voting involves other considerations, such as ensuring that states have the ballot scanners and personnel to conduct signature matching. It will also require printing and mailing ballots before the election and processing them afterward. It is hard to compare which sets of consid-

---

[17] Tim Starks, "Snapshots of How the Pandemic Is Influencing Election Security," *Politico Morning Cybersecurity*, June 8, 2020.

[18] For example, one recent study of five states estimated total costs of between $60 million and $124 million per state to prepare for the election. See Christopher R. Deluzio, Elizabeth Howard, David Levine, Paul Rosenzweig, and Derek Tisler, *Ensuring Safe Elections: Federal Funding Needs for State and Local Governments During the Pandemic*, New York: Brennan Center for Justice, April 30, 2020.

[19] For more information, see Cybersecurity and Infrastructure Security Agency, "#Protect2020," webpage, June 3, 2020.

erations are more difficult to manage; the answer to this could vary by state and by the election processes that each state has in place. In our assessment, we try to identify relevant logistical considerations with each option, but we do not rate their severity on a scale.

There is the separate question of whether considerations across such dimensions as access and integrity might be fundamentally different under pandemic conditions. (They certainly are different for safety and logistics). In terms of access, it seems possible that the benefits of at least remote voting and AVR will be amplified by a pandemic that makes it harder and more dangerous from a public health perspective for people to gather in person. This would be especially true if states had to reduce the number or capacity of polling locations because of pandemic conditions. On the issue of fraud, some critics suggest that an increase in the volume of mail-in ballots could pose a threat to election integrity by overwhelming state officials, creating new opportunities for fraud, or making such processes as signature matching harder to implement.[20] However, there is no evidence that mail-in voting is subject to these threats in the first place, so it seems unlikely that the pandemic itself raises the risk of fraud in a meaningful way. It is true that having a larger number of mail-in ballots will create new demands on election officials, but there is little reason to think that this increase will make it any easier for domestic or foreign actors to perpetrate fraud on a large scale. Safeguards—such as signature matching and, in some places, voter identification requirements—will continue to provide some security, as will the distributed nature of the process. In the following chapters, we discuss some safeguards that are relevant to specific voting options that will continue to secure mail-in voting, even in the face of a pandemic.

In the next chapter, we present each option for voter registration and vote casting and consider its benefits and challenges. We conclude each option's section with an assessment along the four dimensions described, grounding these assessments in the research.

---

[20] Amber Phillips, "Examining the Arguments Against Voting by Mail," *Washington Post*, May 20, 2020. In addition to access and integrity, state officials might wish to consider other factors. For example, there are logistical questions about the time it will take to count and verify a larger number of mail ballots. We do not consider these issues in detail.

CHAPTER FOUR

Evaluation of Options for Registration and Voting During a Pandemic

In this chapter, we evaluate options for registration and voting by providing insights into the four factors already described. Circumstances vary across and even within states, so the factors are discussed generally, but they can be used to inform more-detailed analysis by local election officials and the public. (Our companion report on state laws identifies which categorization a state belongs to in terms of forms of registration and voting.[1]) The options we examine for voter registration are

- in-person registration
- online registration
- mail-in registration.

  For vote casting, we examine

- in-person voting (Election Day and early voting)
- absentee voting and vote-by-mail.

We examine in-person voting for Election Day and early voting together because the factors have similar considerations. We note any differences between them. Similarly, although absentee voting and vote-by-mail are distinct options in terms of their legal basis, they function very similarly and have similar considerations across the factors. Again, we note any differences in the analysis. We also briefly examine

---

[1] Kavanagh et al., 2020.

other forms of remote voting (fax and online) that are likely not feasible for broad use in the fall but have been used for defined populations.

As noted, each state has different laws governing election processes, such as the availability and type of early voting or absentee balloting. Expanding or introducing these options could require legislative action, which might be challenging because most state legislatures usually are only in session for a set number of days each year (and might be even more challenging in an election year). For example, Maryland's General Assembly and Montana's legislature convene for 90 days each year, Wyoming holds just 20 legislative days in even years and 40 in odd years, and Oregon has one of the longest sessions, at 160 days.[2] In some states, a governor can call an emergency session or request one.

Voter Registration

Voter registration options include traditional in-person registration at a government office, such as the DMV or registrar's office; online registration; and mail or phone registration, such as voter registration drives conducted by third parties. To assess the characteristics of safety, integrity, access, and logistics, we draw on available research on in-person, mail-in, and online processes. Most literature on these topics focuses on voting, but we use what research does exist to make inferences that allow us to draw some conclusions on registration.

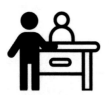

In-Person Registration

In-person registration can refer to AVR (available in 14 states and the District of Columbia) or another dedicated process. As the COVID-19 pandemic gained prominence and states began to implement stay-at-home orders in March 2020, many government agencies, including registrars' offices and DMVs, closed their doors to the public.[3] The

---

[2] National Conference of State Legislatures, "Legislative Session Length," webpage, December 2, 2010.

[3] This occurred in Nevada, which recently implemented AVR. Associated Press, "Voter Registrations Slow with Virus Closing DMV Offices," *US News and World Report*, April 2, 2020.

reopening process has varied across and within states in terms of timing and conditions, including considerations for how government agencies resume operations and serving the public.

Safety

As an in-person process, this type of registration will face several safety challenges in a pandemic context. Providing a safe environment for in-person registration, whether at a county clerk's office, at the DMV, or at other government offices will require implementing safe practices, such as social distancing to spread out lines, using protective equipment (for example, plexiglass dividers at service counters), and sanitizing materials.[4] High-touch surfaces, such as screens that use styluses or computer keyboards, will also need to be cleaned regularly, and workers will need to have PPE to safely handle documents, such as personal identification or other paperwork required for a prospective voter to establish residency. Some locations might relax these safety requirements as the threat from COVID-19 dissipates but should be ready to reinforce those regulations in the event of potential continuing cases. Overall, in-person registration will require safety constraints, but these can be mitigated somewhat with precautions.

Integrity

In-person registration, particularly when accomplished at the same time as registering for other government services (for example, driver's license, public assistance), often involves providing proof of residency; three states require proof of citizenship to register (Alabama, Arizona, and Georgia).[5] All states require a signed attestation of citizenship when registering to vote, which usually carries a warning about the

---

[4] Guidance on best practices for preventing the spread of COVID-19 is available from the Centers for Disease Control and Prevention, "How to Protect Yourself & Others," webpage, April 24, 2020a.

[5] VoteRiders, "What's the Difference Between Voter ID and Voter Registration?" webpage, undated. Kansas's citizenship requirement was struck down by the 10th Federal Circuit Court of Appeals. See "Court Says Kansas Can't Require Voters to Show Citizenship Proof," PBS Newshour website, April 29, 2020.

penalties for fraudulent registration.[6] As a result, the process is typically secure and identity verification is possible. Implementing social distancing and other safety procedures, such as barriers between stations, can also promote privacy to some extent for those registering in person because it reduces the opportunities for others to see the information being provided (for example, date of birth, social security number). In terms of voting registration eligibility concerns, noncitizen voting registration might occur more frequently than ineligible voting registration of those with felony records (ineligible based on state laws). There have been instances of registrations for noncitizens and other errors as states have implemented AVR (California experienced several problems in 2018), but these have been identified and corrected.[7]

Access

Safe access to in-person registration under COVID-19 conditions is likely not equally distributed across groups. States might need to consider extending operating hours or reserving time for vulnerable populations (for example, the elderly or immunocompromised) to provide safe access. Alternatively, election officials could examine opening temporary registration centers, such as drive-through options or other facilities, to provide access while implementing safety measures. Persons with disabilities might require additional accommodation, which most state agencies are already prepared to provide because of the requirements of the Americans with Disabilities Act.[8] The implications for access are likely to depend somewhat on the specific registration process used. For example, an in-person system that requires someone to complete a separate registration process might create several hurdles to access, such as the need to go to a registration site. However, an in-person automatic system, such as AVR, can increase access by reducing

---

[6] This applies to contests for federal office. Some jurisdictions allow noncitizens to vote in local elections.

[7] Matt Vasilogambros, "Glitches in California Embolden Automatic Voter Registration Foes," *Stateline*, October 17, 2019.

[8] U.S. Department of Justice, "A Guide to Disability Rights Laws," webpage, February 2020a.

impediments—for example, by making registration an opt-out process and combining it with another transaction.[9]

Logistics

All states provide in-person registration, including through the local registrar's office and other government agencies, such as the DMV. Several logistical considerations will have to be made when implementing additional safety measures. First, officials will need to ensure an adequate supply of PPE, protective items in the workplace, and sanitation supplies and services. This can also mean purchasing disposable items, such as single-use pens or films for screens that customers use once and are then replaced. Officials will also need to ensure social distancing, which could require longer hours, more employees, or more locations (including temporary facilities) where people can register. Finally, officials will need to communicate changes to affected populations, including through mailers and online outlets (for example, official websites, social media). Election officials will want to ensure that prospective voters are not inadvertently discouraged from registering because they are unaware of changes to office hours or because of longer lines than usual.

The scramble to procure PPE, protective screens, and other equipment in spring 2020 indicates that state and local election officials need to plan early—projecting the number of people they expect to want to register in the run-up to the general election. Adapting government offices to ensure social distancing and protect workers requires time to plan and implement. There will be additional costs to adapt workspaces for protection and to ensure social distancing, which could include markings on floors, additional signage, and personnel to remind the public of the additional requirements. Election workers also might fall ill and need temporary replacements, who could be other employees or trained volunteers (where allowed).

The main cost considerations are

---

[9] Kevin Morris and Peter Dunphy, *AVR Impact on State Voter Registration*, New York: Brennan Center for Justice, 2019. Morris and Dunphy note increases in voter registrations, whereas the analysis of McGhee and Romero, 2020, indicates uneven experience across states adopting AVR.

- PPE, sanitation supplies, and single-use items
- new office layouts, including protective barriers and notices (for example, floor markings)
- additional labor costs for extending hours, managing customer flow, or staffing temporary facilities
- rental costs for temporary facilities, if used
- mailing and other communication costs to inform the public
- additional janitorial services.

Summary

In-person voter registration could be particularly complicated in the fall if continued or renewed pandemic conditions lead to further closures of government offices, thereby restricting access for voters wishing to register to vote. Implementing safety procedures (for example, the use of appointments to manage the number of people in any one place at a given time) can reduce the risk of transmission of the virus but can also lead to increased waiting times and reduced capacity. This runs the risk of preventing some potential voters from registering, particularly if they give up on the process or are deterred from trying in the first place. In-person voter registration, on the other hand, allows for processing documentation that proves residency, notifying registrants of the penalties for fraudulent registration, and addressing errors or misunderstandings, so integrity concerns might be lower.

Online Registration

As of June 2020, 38 states and the District of Columbia offered online voter registration, and Oklahoma was in the process of implementing a full system.[10] Several states have also worked to ensure that online registration is optimized for use on mobile devices, such as smartphones, and to provide accessibility to non-English speakers.[11] Information requirements vary from state to state for online registration: Some

---

[10] National Conference of State Legislatures, 2020b.

[11] Pew Charitable Trusts, "Online Voter Registration: Trends in Development and Implementation," May 2015, p. 4.

only require a date of birth and zip code; others require date of birth, a valid identification number (for example, driver's license) and full Social Security number. Figure 4.1 shows which states have online registration and/or AVR.

Safety

Online registration promotes safety because it does not require any face-to-face contact with a registering official. A prospective voter accesses an online form, fills in the requested information, and submits it through the web portal for review and entry into the voter reg-

Figure 4.1
States with Online Registration and Automatic Voter Registration

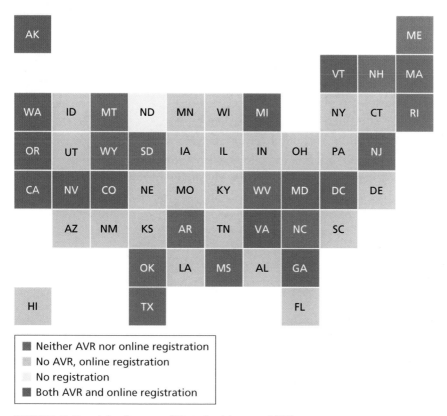

Neither AVR nor online registration
No AVR, online registration
No registration
Both AVR and online registration

SOURCE: National Conference of State Legislatures, 2020b.

istration database. Some voters might not have regular access to the internet, so this approach would require them to find public computers (for example, at a local library) to complete the process. Because online registration should be a remote process for most, there are few safety considerations.

Integrity

Online voter registration has to have a process for verifying the registrant's identity and for providing secure transmission of personal information. Even with such systems, this approach could have a higher integrity risk than an in-person process. The primary method states use to authenticate a registrant is requesting a driver's license number or information from another form of government-issued identification and checking this information against the relevant database. To protect voter information confidentiality, registration websites should provide for encrypted submission of information and implement other security features, such as multiple screens to capture individual pieces of information and use of captcha forms to prevent automated attempts to register.[12] Privacy and security can also be affected if someone uses a public computer (for example, at a library). As noted earlier, research suggests that the risk of fraud with online and other remote processes is slightly higher than in-person processes but still extremely low.[13] However, there might be other security considerations associated with foreign or other interference, such as an adversary manipulating vulnerabilities in the public-facing website to gain access to a back-end database.

Access

In general, as a remote process, online registration could increase access among those for whom registering in person is a deterrent, especially in a pandemic context. However, online registration will also create some new hurdles. First, online registration will need to accommodate persons with disabilities, non-English speakers, and those with no permanent residence. Second, most online voter registration processes require

---

[12] National Conference of State Legislatures, 2020b.

[13] This finding has been confirmed by multiple analyses. See Goel et al., 2020; Minnite and Callahan, 2003; Reality Check Team, 2020; Stein, 2003; and Viesbeck, 2020.

people to have a state-issued identification, such as a driver's license, to verify the voter.[14] This means that those who do not already have such identification would have to register in person, which can pose an access constraint for some populations, such as those who live far away from a state agency or those who have long-term illnesses. There is limited research on the scope of this constraint, although it is worth noting that identification requirements for voting processes appear to have only a small negative effect on turnout. We can infer that the effect on access to registration also might be minor.[15]

Third, a significant hurdle for some populations (for example, low-income households) is reasonable access to online resources, both in terms of an end point (such as a computer, laptop, smartphone, or tablet) and network access. Some populations that would use other publicly available resources, such as public libraries, could face barriers to registration if these facilities are not open.

For those with a smartphone or tablet but no regular internet access, open Wi-Fi at public offices or other spaces is an option—but one that carries significant cybersecurity risk given the potential for a hacker to steal confidential information or to execute a man-in-the-middle attack that alters the transmitted information or diverts it from the intended destination.

Overall, then, the effect of online registration on access might be mixed. Although it can increase access for some populations, new requirements (such as access to Wi-Fi or possession of identification) could create new obstacles for some voters.

Logistics

Developing and implementing an online voter registration system is not a simple task and requires careful planning and implementation to ensure that government agencies have the systems and processes in place to process the information. In many states with online registration, the prospective voter might start at the state election director's website and then be directed to the local jurisdiction for the initial sub-

---

[14] National Conference of State Legislatures, 2020b.

[15] Hajnal, Lajevardi, and Nielson, 2017; Highton, 2017.

mission of registration information. This information has to be validated and transmitted, preferably electronically, for inclusion in the voter registration database. Pew found in research on the implementation of online voter registration that the costs are modest, ranging from approximately $100,000 to more than $1.4 million per state.[16] These costs might not always account for staff time, software validation and verification, training, or communicating the process and requirements to the public.

In states where local jurisdictions have more autonomy in administering systems (such as bottom-up voter registration systems), there might be issues related to implementing common data formats. Something as simple as the date format (month-day-year versus day-month-year) can lead to discrepancies or errors if there is variation across jurisdictions. States implementing online registration have to account for these requirements, including testing and validation of software prior to going "live."

The main cost considerations are

- software development, testing, and deployment costs
- staff training
- mailer and other communication costs to raise public awareness.

Summary
Implementing a new process and system is a challenge in the best of circumstances, but in an environment of compressed timelines and urgency, errors and security vulnerabilities can arise unnoticed. Online registration requires controls to ensure secure entry and transmission of personal information, prevent hijacking of web sessions, and counter the (relatively low) risk of fraud through registration of false personas or registering people in multiple jurisdictions. The Electronic Registration Information Center, a nonprofit organization that manages a system for checking and validating voter registration records across 30 member states and the District of Columbia, helps reduce

---

[16] Pew Charitable Trusts, 2015, p. 5.

the instances of deliberate or inadvertent duplicate registrations (for example, for when someone moves to a new state).[17]

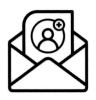

Mail-In Registration

Although in-person and online voter registration are the most common forms of registration, there is also mail-in registration. Voters in most states can use the National Mail Voter Registration Form available from the U.S. Election Assistance Commission or mail-in forms from their state or local jurisdictions.[18] The national form is available in 15 languages and accepted by all states except North Dakota and Wyoming. (It is also not accepted in the U.S. territories of Puerto Rico, the Virgin Islands, American Samoa, and Guam.) New Hampshire only accepts the form as a request for an absentee ballot. Many states and jurisdictions have their own registration forms available for download online.[19] Voters eligible under UOCAVA must use a separate process and form.[20]

Safety

Mail-in voter registration is largely safe because it is a one-way transaction (if current understanding of COVID-19 is correct and transmission on paper surfaces is not a primary risk).[21] Voters can download and

---

[17] Electronic Registration Information Center, homepage, undated.

[18] See U.S. Election Assistance Commission, "National Mail Voter Registration Form," webpage, undated-a.

[19] For example, Mississippi, New Jersey, and Washington all provide forms for each county in the state. Cook County, Illinois, also provides forms. See Cook County Clerk's Office, "Register to Vote," webpage, undated; State of Mississippi, "Mississippi Mail-In Voter Registration Application," online form, undated; New Jersey Division of Elections, "Register to Vote!" webpage, June 16, 2020; and Washington State, "Elections," webpage, undated.

[20] Federal Voting Assistance Program, "Voter Registration and Ballots," webpages for military and overseas citizens, undated-c.

[21] Tara Parker-Pope, "What's the Risk of Catching Coronavirus from a Surface?" *New York Times*, June 3, 2020. There is still uncertainty over the viability of COVID-19 on different surfaces, but one preliminary study found that it deteriorated faster on cardboard than on other surfaces (the study did not specifically examine paper). See Neeltje van Doremale, Trenton Bushmaker, Dylan H. Morris, Myndi G. Holbrook, Amandine

fill in forms themselves or receive forms from party representatives or other individuals engaged in voter registration drives. Receiving a form from third parties does increase the potential for transmission because it involves interaction with another person (although social distancing measures can be used, such as leaving forms in mailboxes). Still, elections staff will require PPE to process the paper unless other steps are taken, such as storing mail-in forms for several days, but these timelines also have to account for registration deadlines in states that have them.

Integrity

Although the risk is low, mail-in registration presents some increased risk for fraudulent registration (for example, someone seeking to register multiple times or in the wrong jurisdiction or a noncitizen seeking to register). However, this risk is largely mitigated with additional safeguards (for example, requiring registrants to attest that they are eligible to vote and acknowledge the potential for prosecution) and verification processes carried out by jurisdictions and states. The Heritage Foundation's database of voter fraud cases documents 162 counts of false registration from 1982 to 2020.[22] Privacy, on the other hand, is heightened because the information provided during the transaction (including personal information and party affiliation) is known only to the applicant and to the registrar processing the request.[23] States that allow registration by mail often require a copy of the voter's identification as an additional

---

Gamble, Brandi Williamson, Azaibi Tamin, Jennifer L. Harcourt, Natalie J. Thornburg, Susan I. Gerber, James O. Lloyd-Smith, Emmei de Wit, and Vincent Munster, "Aerosol and Surface Stability of SARS-CoV-2 as Compared with SARS-CoV-1," *New England Journal of Medicine*, Vol. 382, No. 16, March 2020.

[22] According to our analysis of the Heritage Foundation Election Fraud databases, several cases of election fraud consist of multiple counts (e.g., false registration and fraudulent use of absentee ballots). We have broken these cases out to account for cases of specific types of fraud. Heritage notes that its database is not comprehensive and does not include cases that were not fully investigated. Heritage Foundation, "A Sampling of Recent Election Fraud Cases from Across the United States," database, undated.

[23] Some information—such as voter names, addresses, and party affiliation—are made available through the voter file. States vary in terms of who is able to request copies of the voter file and which information is releasable. See National Conference of State Legislatures, "Access to and Use of Voter Registration Lists," webpage, August 5, 2019a.

check on voter fraud. In some cases, a voter needing assistance to fill in the registration form might be required to note that someone assisted the voter. There is some potential for undue influence, such as threatening someone to keep them from registering, forcing them to register against their will, or falsely registering by posing as family members. In general, however, what research exists suggests that although there might be a slight increase in the risk to integrity from a mail-in process compared with an in-person one, it is likely to be low overall.[24]

Access

Voters have several options for getting a mail-in registration form, including downloading a form from their local registrar's office, using the National Mail Voter Registration Form where allowed, and through voter registration drives. The national form is available in 15 languages, but persons requiring special accommodation might need assistance in filling out the form. The 1984 Voting Accessibility for the Elderly and Handicapped Act requires providing assistance to the disabled and elderly for registration and voting in federal elections.[25] Some states require copies of identification to confirm eligibility, which can disadvantage individuals who do not have identification and those without easy access to printers, scanners, or copiers, although these might be available at low or no cost at libraries and post offices.[26] States and local jurisdictions also might have their own forms available from official election websites. Overall, what research exists on mail-in processes like voting and registration suggests that these processes can have a positive net effect on access, and that even identification requirements could have less of a negative effect than is sometimes assumed. However, it is also worth noting that implications might not be equally distributed across demographic groups.[27]

---

[24] Stein, 2013; Goel et al., 2020.

[25] 52 U.S. Code Ch. 201, Voting Accessibility for the Elderly and Handicapped.

[26] This group typically includes such nondrivers as younger populations or seniors whose licenses might have expired or who are no longer able to drive.

[27] Karp and Banducci, 2000; Southwell and Burchett, 2000.

Logistics

Increasing mail-in registration requires planning for hand-processing or investing in automated processing to handle larger volumes of registration forms. Mail-in registration forms are either printed by the registrant or provided through government agencies, political parties, or other third parties. The forms have to be received and processed in line with state deadlines for voter registration.

Processing paper forms can be time-consuming and can lead to errors if data entry is by hand or optical scanning does not recognize or process handwriting correctly. Election officials might need to plan out processes to address identification of such errors and take corrective action, including contacting voters, in a timely manner. The costs for handling mail-in registration could include additional training for personnel, hiring temporary workers or recruiting additional volunteers, and providing for chain of custody on registration materials, including safe and secure storage.

Potential voters also should be made aware (1) of legal deadlines for registering where applicable and (2) that mail-in registration forms might be delayed in processing by the U.S. Postal Service. Deadlines for receiving and processing registrations could prove challenging to accommodate all the prospective voters if there are delays in receipt of registration applications or to address errors.

The main cost considerations are

- printing and mailing costs for forms
- mail-processing equipment (letter openers, sorters)
- processing equipment to scan returned forms
- staff costs for hand-sorting and/or data entry (normally for smaller jurisdictions).

Summary

Mail-in registration is relatively safe from physical health threats but might raise some risks in terms of integrity and access. It can also create a potentially high logistical burden for election officials. This might be especially true as the deadline for registration or Election Day approaches, particularly if election officials need to contact voters for corrective actions. Handling large volumes of paper registration forms can also lead to errors in transferring information to electronic files.

Summary of Evaluation of Options for Voter Registration

Table 4.1 summarizes the options for voter registration, along with the considerations and level of risk for each. We do not include considerations that apply equally to all options—for example, all options must provide accommodations for non-English speakers and voters with disabilities. As noted previously, our assessments are based on existing empirical evidence about the effects of different voting policies and processes on access and integrity and an assessment of the safety and logistical implications in the context of a pandemic.

The most useful way to consider these assessments is in relative terms. Table 4.1 suggests that risks associated with safety (specifically that associated with physical health related to COVID-19) is highest for in-person registration. On access, risk is highest for in-person registration because of the requirement that an eligible voter travel to another location, somewhat lower for online registration, and lowest for mail-in registration. However, it is also worth noting that AVR,

Table 4.1
Summary of Risks for Implementing Voter Registration Options During a Pandemic

	Risks to Safety	Risks to Integrity	Risks to Access	Logistical Considerations
In-person	High • New interpersonal contact • Automatic voter registration (AVR) could reduce risk	Minimal	Moderate • Travel required	Safety and sanitation mitigations • Communication • Training
Online	Minimal	Low (but higher than in-person) • Cybersecurity	Low • Internet availability • Technology requirements	Online system, processing • Verification • Training • Communication
Mail-in	Minimal	Low (but higher than in-person)	Minimal	Processing and verification • Training • Verification

which might occur in person, can perhaps increase access and reduce this risk by conducting registration as part of another process (despite being conducted in person).[28] Integrity-related risk is low across the board but slightly higher for remote options. However, all options have significant logistical considerations. For in-person registration, logistical considerations focus on safety. For online and mail-in options, the logistical considerations are largely focused on creating systems to support remote processes and acquiring the equipment needed for processing submitted registrations. It would be difficult to rank options based on the severity of logistical concerns. Each option has different risks on this dimension, but they are not clearly more or less than other options. Considering across options, if all risks are assessed to be equal, risk seems relatively lower, at least in the pandemic context we focus on here, for online and mail-in options than for in-person options. However, it is worth emphasizing that a given state is unlikely to rank these four dimensions equally; each will have its own priorities and constraints (political and legal) and will choose those options that are the best fit for its needs.

Voting

In this section, we address the different options for voting:

- in-person, on Election Day or early voting
- absentee voting or vote-by-mail
- remote voting (for example, email or web-based voting, fax).

We address in-person voting on Election Day and early voting together and note where there are variations. Similarly, although absentee voting and vote-by-mail are distinct from a legal standpoint, they function similarly and we address them together while noting any differences.

---

[28] Franklin and Grier, 1997; Knack, 1995.

In-Person Voting (Election Day or Early Voting)
Safety

Voting in person, whether on Election Day or earlier, has significant safety implications within a pandemic context because pollworkers need to account for the safety of both the voting public and themselves (see Figure 4.2). This can involve providing for social distancing, limiting the number of people waiting in enclosed spaces, and ensuring safety at check-in and in the voting booth.[29] It also means having necessary PPE and sanitation supplies, including for individuals who might arrive without their own. In some jurisdictions, the process of making choices on a ballot is separate from the physical vote casting, which can involve scanning a ballot into a separate machine or feeding a ballot into a ballot box.[30] During the primary elections that occurred after the introduction of pandemic restrictions, several states (Wisconsin is one example) experienced problems with providing enough pollworkers at precincts (many workers backed out because of COVID-19 fears), which led to a reduced number of polling places being open.[31] For the April 28, 2020, primary in Ohio, in-person voting was restricted to registrars' offices and only open to voters requiring special

Figure 4.2
In-Person Voting During a Pandemic

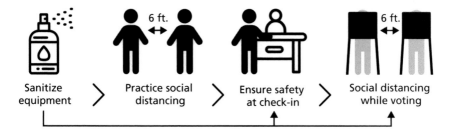

| Sanitize equipment | | Practice social distancing | | Ensure safety at check-in | | Social distancing while voting |

---

[29] Centers for Disease Control and Prevention, "Social Distancing," webpage, May 6, 2020c.

[30] For the types of voting equipment used in each U.S. state and county, see Verified Voting, "The Verifier—Polling Place Equipment—November 2020," webpage, undated.

[31] Alison Dirr and Mary Spicuzza, "What We Know So Far About Why Milwaukee Only Had 5 Voting Sites for Tuesday's Election While Madison Had 66," *Milwaukee Journal Sentinel*, April 9, 2020.

accommodations or who did not have a permanent residence to receive an absentee ballot.[32] In the fall, state and local officials might expect a larger turnout for the general election and opt to have most—preferably all—voting places open. Some voting precincts, however, might not have enough physical space to allow for adequate social distancing (that is, room to space out lines and to provide separation between voting machines). This can create access issues and risks as well.

Voting precincts will need to have appropriate PPE and sanitizing agents. The three primary voting equipment vendors in the United States—ES&S, Dominion, and Hart InterCivic—have issued guidance on sanitizing procedures.[33] In places where voting machines cannot be spaced far enough apart, officials will have to determine whether additional shielding, such as plexiglass, is needed. In many jurisdictions, pollworkers are volunteers and more than half are over the age of 60. The Centers for Disease Control and Prevention has indicated that people over the age of 65 have a higher risk of developing more-serious complications from COVID-19 than the general population.[34] Election officials will also need to consider how to screen pollworkers for symptoms of COVID-19 and plan for contingencies where some pollworkers might need to be sent home.

Some voters invariably need extra assistance on Election Day because they are either unfamiliar with the voting equipment or might make errors that lead to a spoiled ballot. Procedures for these circumstances should be in place, and pollworkers will need training on how to safely assist voters and ensure their right to vote. Pollworkers will also need to have extra PPE on hand for voters who arrive at the polling place without a mask, and they will need training and guidance on how to handle situations in which a prospective voter refuses to

---

[32] Rick Rouan, "Here's What You Need to Know About Ohio's Delayed Primary Election," *Columbus Dispatch*, April 26, 2020.

[33] U.S. Election Assistance Commission, "Vendor and Manufacturer Guidance on Cleaning Voting Machines and Other Election Technology," webpage, undated-b.

[34] For pollworker demographics, see Matt Vasilogambros, "Few People Want to Be Poll Workers, and That's a Problem," *Stateline*, October 22, 2018. On the higher risks that older people face, see Centers for Disease Control and Prevention, "Older Adults," webpage, April 30, 2020b.

comply with guidelines, which could be voluntary in some locations but required in others.

Early voting seeks to spread out voter demand by providing more opportunities to vote in person before Election Day; this, in turn, might reduce the amount of time people have to wait in line on any given day and reduce the number of people in a polling place at the same time. For those who still wish to vote on Election Day, early voting also could result in shorter lines because other voters already voted.

To summarize, although the safety implications of any in-person voting process will be significant (especially where turnout is high), implementing early voting—especially for an extended period at a wide variety of locations—can mitigate some of these safety implications.

Integrity

In-person voting, whether early or on Election Day, has strong protections against challenges to election integrity. There are 36 states with some form of voter identification requirement, although the enforcement of those requirements varies from state to state.[35] In some states, the requirement is strict, in that voters have to show identification; if they cannot, they must provide identification within a set time frame after casting a provisional ballot. Other states request a form of identification but will allow for attestation of the right to vote and provision of information to establish identity (for example, address, date of birth). Other states use signature matching, an affidavit attesting to eligibility (with associated penalties for falsely attesting), and/or providing personal information (such as the last four digits of one's Social Security number) to establish voter identity.[36] However, it is worth noting that the overall risk of fraud is low, so these additional verification measures might have only a marginal effect on election integrity (and, as noted previously, no real effect on perceptions of integrity).[37]

---

[35] Wendy Underhill, "Voter Identification Requirements: Voter ID Laws," National Conference of State Legislatures webpage, February 24, 2020.

[36] National Conference of State Legislatures, "Voter Verification Without ID Documents," webpage, undated.

[37] Charles Stewart III, Stephen Ansolabehere, and Nathaniel Persily, "Revisiting Public Opinion on Voter Identification and Voter Fraud in an Era of Increasing Partisan Polarization," *Stanford Law Review*, Vol. 68, 2016, p. 1455.

Secret ballots are supported through voting booths or stations that provide voters privacy when making the choices and casting their ballot. Privacy is reinforced by social distancing and spacing voting machines farther apart. Some voters might need assistance in filling in or casting their ballots, which can decrease privacy. Polling places have restrictions on active campaigning or advocacy in or near the voting booth to miti-gate against undue influence. Although voters can choose to have some-one accompany them to assist with voting, to prevent undue influence, that person cannot be the voter's employer or an agent acting on behalf of the employer or a union.[38] According to the Heritage Foundation voter fraud database, there have been 25 counts of polling-place fraud involv-ing either impersonation or illegal assistance from 1982 to 2020, which covers documented cases the researchers were able to identify.[39]

Access

As officials plan for in-person voting, they will need to address the requirements for accessibility. There will be some access concerns asso-ciated directly with the pandemic itself (for example, disrupted public transportation or parents with child care issues). Promoting access for all voters requires providing polling places that are sufficient to meet demand and geographically distributed to support all communities. This might be a challenge, given the need for locations with enough space to allow social distancing and the need to recruit enough pollworkers. Several states and jurisdictions (for example, Los Angeles County and Texas) have implemented voting center models that allow them to reduce the number of physical precincts while serving the same populations, but there is evidence that this change can adversely affect some popula-tions, particularly those that end up having to travel farther (which can be particularly burdensome for those who do not have work flexibility

---

[38] U.S. Department of Justice, "Statutes Enforced by the Voting Section," webpage, March 11, 2020b.

[39] The Heritage Foundation defines *illegal assistance* as "forcing or intimidating voters—particularly the elderly, disabled, illiterate, and those for whom English is a second language—to vote for particular candidates while supposedly providing them with 'assistance'" (Heritage Foundation, undated).

on Election Day).[40] The concept of a voting center is intended to allow voters to find the most convenient place to vote rather than tying them to a specific precinct near their residence that they might not be able to access on Election Day. In addition to the number of polling places per capita, there is also the question of polling place "quality," encompassing how well advertised the location is, the physical state of the building (for example, adequate lighting and access to restrooms), and the availability of parking or public transit.[41] Recent studies indicate that minorities are more likely to face longer lines at polling places, which can dissuade voters who have less flexible work schedules or cause them to grow frustrated and leave without voting.[42]

There will also be accessibility issues not related to the pandemic that are relevant across elections. Safety measures (such as greater distances between check-in areas and voting machines) at individual polling places could improve accessibility for individuals with disabilities, but some jurisdictions also might reduce the number of polling places open on Election Day because of potentially reduced pollworker availability and the unsuitability of some previously used locations. Prior studies have shown that voter turnout rates are lower among persons with disabilities, particularly those who report having difficulty traveling outside their homes or driving.[43] The forms of difficulty include trouble using voting equipment, waiting in line for long periods, finding a polling place, and getting in. Many jurisdictions have worked

---

[40] Jeronimo Cortina and Brandon Rottinghaus, "'The Quiet Revolution': Convenience Voting, Vote Centers, and Turnout in Texas Elections," conference paper presented to the Election Sciences, Reform, and Administration Conference, University of Pennsylvania, 2019. Los Angeles's experience is too recent to evaluate the impact on different communities.

[41] For an examination of polling place quality across ethnic and income lines, see Matt A. Barreto, Mara Cohen-Marks, and Nathan D. Woods, "Are All Precincts Created Equal? The Prevalence of Low-Quality Precincts in Low-Income and Minority Communities," *Political Research Quarterly*, Vol. 62, No. 3, September 2009.

[42] Daniel Garisto, "Smartphone Data Show Voters in Black Neighborhoods Wait Longer," *Scientific American*, October 1, 2019. Also see Hannah Klain, Kevin Morris, Max Feldman, and Rebecca Ayala, *Waiting to Vote: Racial Disparities in Election Day Experiences*, New York: Brennan Center for Justice, June 3, 2020.

[43] Lisa Schur, Mason Ameri, and Meera Adya, "Disability, Voter Turnout, and Polling Place Accessibility," *Social Science Quarterly*, Vol. 98, No. 5, November 2017.

to address these issues (for example, by providing assistive devices for voting machines and allowing curbside ballot drop-off or voting for those unable to enter the polling place).[44]

Early voting expands opportunities for other populations, such as those who work long hours on Election Day and find it difficult to get to the polls during the day. Early voting often involves fewer polling places during the early voting period than are available on Election Day, and election officials need to evaluate their distribution and availability to serve voting populations. Although early voting can support social distancing by allowing voters to spread out over time and locations, the empirical evidence that exists suggests that the effects of early voting on turnout are less clear. Most studies find only a small effect in terms of bringing in new voters, although it might increase convenience for those who intended to vote anyway.[45]

Logistics

Election officials will have to plan for identifying and approving potentially new polling places that can accommodate greater social distancing and allow for installing other protective barriers. Some traditional voting locations, such as retirement homes, will likely be deemed unsuitable from a public health perspective because they expose vulnerable populations, while others might not be large enough. Schools are often used as polling places and, although the risk to children from COVID-19 is believed to be lower (noting that some children have experienced severe complications known as *multisystem inflammatory syndrome*), election officials might need to consider ways to minimize the interaction between voters and the school population on Election Day.[46] Planning will need to address controlling the flow of voters to promote social distancing and ordering adequate supplies of PPE, sanitizing agents, and cleaning cloths. Some voters might come to the polls

---

[44] Schur, Ameri, and Adya, 2017, pp. 1379–1381; Tetsuya Matsubayashi and Michiko Ueda, "Disability and Voting," *Disability and Health Journal*, Vol. 7, 2014.

[45] For example, see Gronke, Galanes-Rosenbaum, and Miller, 2007; Stein, 1998.

[46] Harvard Medical School, "Coronavirus Outbreak and Kids," June 11, 2020.

without face coverings, and election officials will need to have extras on hand, otherwise they risk turning voters away for health reasons.

Election officials will need to plan for ordering additional supplies and equipment, identifying and reviewing polling places, recruiting pollworkers, and setting up equipment that might take longer than usual. The costs associated with additional safety protocols could include purchasing additional equipment, providing training for pollworkers, holding recruitment drives to identify pollworkers, and implementing procedures to ensure proper handling of voting materials.

Early voting will also need to have measures in place for secure overnight storage of voting equipment and materials. Planning for early voting might require longer timelines to review existing early voting places for suitability, identify new facilities and negotiate access, order materials, and recruit pollworkers and train them on new procedures.

The main cost considerations are

- PPE, sanitation supplies, and one-time-use items
- new polling place layouts, including protective barriers and notices (for example, floor markings and signage)
- pollworker recruitment and training costs
- mailing and other communication costs to inform the public
- additional janitorial services.

Summary

In-person voting could present significant challenges if demand from voters remains high despite concerns over COVID-19 and if the supply of pollworkers is constrained. Enforcing social distancing requirements will be difficult, and pollworkers might have to engage with voters who refuse to comply with health safety requirements, potentially endangering pollworkers and other voters. Safety concerns related to physical health are perhaps the most significant, but there are also logistical and access considerations. By providing an opportunity to space out the demand for in-person voting and relieve stress on Election Day, early voting can mitigate some safety concerns but does not eliminate them. However, even early voting entails risks that the demand will cluster closer to Election Day, particularly in jurisdictions that have less experience with early voting.

Absentee Voting and Vote-by-Mail

Every state has some form of absentee voting, and 14 states have some form of vote-by-mail (see Figure 4.3). For absentee ballots, the requirements vary on whether an excuse is required and what reasons qualify a voter to vote by mail. As of June 2020, 16 states required an excuse to receive an absentee ballot, 21 allowed absentee balloting without requiring an excuse (hereafter referred to as *no-excuse absentee*), seven states and the District of Columbia had no-excuse absentee balloting with a permanent mail-in option, and one (Pennsylvania) required an excuse for an absentee ballot while also having a mail-in option.[47] Five states have universal vote-by-mail (Colorado, Hawaii, Oregon, Utah, and Washington).

Some states implemented emergency measures for their primaries to make absentee ballots more broadly available. Connecticut, for example, normally requires an excuse to qualify for an absentee ballot. Governor Ned Lamont issued an executive order for the August 11

Figure 4.3
Processes for Mail-In Ballots

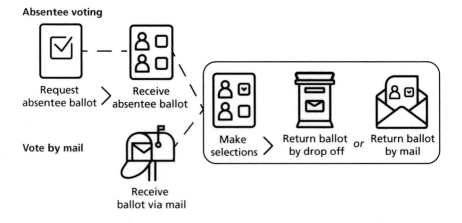

---

[47] Kavanagh et al, 2020.

primary that sought to cover the pandemic as a qualifying "illness" (even for those who did not have the virus) as long as no federally approved vaccine is available. Applying this standard for the general election, however, will require legislative action.[48] Other states, such as Michigan, have sent all registered voters absentee ballot request forms to prompt voters to consider this option.[49]

Safety

As a remote process, safety concerns about absentee voting are minimal. Absentee voting, regardless of whether an excuse is required to receive a ballot, and vote-by-mail provide a safe separation of the voter from others when deciding and casting the ballot.[50] Voters request absentee ballots and receive them at their home address of record, where they can make their choices and return the completed ballot to a drop-box or polling place or through the mail. If voters choose to deliver their ballots through an in-person process, however, this can undermine safety gains that come from remote voting. Other methods of remote voting maintain separation and thus more completely reduce health risks. Pollworkers and election officials can safeguard themselves by wearing PPE while processing returned ballots and practicing social distancing whenever possible.

Integrity

Voters using an absentee ballot or vote-by-mail have to attest to the integrity of the ballot through a variety of methods. Eight states and the District of Columbia require only a signed statement; 30 use signature matching to check that the person casting the ballot is the same person who registered, although there are potential issues with accurately matching signatures that change over time. Twelve states require additional measures, such as a witness's signature to accompany a signed statement (four states), signature matching and a witness's sig-

---

[48] Mark Pazniokas and Ana Radelat, "On Easing Absentee Voting, Connecticut Looks to November and Beyond," *CT Mirror*, May 23, 2020.

[49] Paul Steinhauser, "Michigan Says All Voters Will Be Sent Absentee Ballot Applications," Fox News, May 19, 2020.

[50] van Doremale et al., 2020; Parker-Pope, 2020.

nature (four states), or a notarized affidavit (four states). Three states (Alabama, Arkansas, and Missouri) require voters to also submit copies of their identification.[51] Even with these additional measures, voting by mail is often criticized as increasing the risk of fraud. Analysis suggests that rates of fraud are very low overall. Although they are slightly higher for remote voting than in-person voting, they can remain very low overall if appropriate safeguards, such as signature verification, are implemented.[52] The Heritage Foundation database of voter fraud cases documents 174 counts of fraudulent use of absentee or vote-by-mail ballots from 1982 to 2020 across the United States, although this again represents only documented cases. Multiple other analyses find low incidence of fraud across mail-in voting types.[53] Large-scale fraud would be very difficult to conduct, given measures to secure and account for every ballot. Ballots are laid out at the jurisdiction and state level, leading to variations across jurisdictions that an adversary would have to copy. In addition to signature matching, ballots are barcoded so that election officials and voters can track them, and the U.S. Postal Service also offers smart tracking for election mail.[54]

Absentee ballots and vote-by-mail promote privacy for voters, who can fill in ballots in their homes and insert them into privacy sleeves before placing them in an envelope. States vary in the rules they have in place for who can return an absentee ballot: Most will allow a family member or a designated agent to return the ballot on the voter's behalf; several do not specify a restriction; Alabama allows only the voter to do

---

[51] National Conference of State Legislatures, "Verification of Absentee Ballots," webpage, January 21, 2020a. Also see Missouri Secretary of State, "How to Vote," webpage, undated.

[52] Commission on Federal Election Reform, *Building Confidence in U.S. Elections: Report of The Commission on Federal Election Reform*, September 2005, p. 35; Minnite and Callahan, 2003; Reality Check Team, 2020; Jason Snead, *The Unnecessary Risks of Mandated and Rushed Vote-by-Mail*, Honest Elections Project, July 2020.

[53] Heritage Foundation, undated; Reality Check Team, 2020.

[54] U.S. Postal Service, "Election Mail," webpage, undated. See also Center for Civic Design, *Design Documentation: Vote-by-Mail Envelope Design for California*, Omaha, Neb.: Oxide Design Co, December 15, 2017.

so.[55] There is still potential for undue influence on the voter outside the voting place, such as someone paying or otherwise forcing the voter to make specific choices. There are 64 documented counts of vote-buying in the Heritage Foundation database from 1982 to 2020, but as before the database does not claim to be comprehensive.[56] Overall, although the risk to integrity might be higher for mail-in voting than for in-person voting, the baseline risk of fraud is low across options.

Access

Existing empirical evidence on mail-in voting suggests that, on balance, this method appears to increase access and turnout by removing some hurdles to voting (for example, getting to the polls, waiting in lines).[57] However, the effect is modest in size and can be offset by other access considerations. Absentee ballots and vote-by-mail need to address several access issues, such as accommodating non-English speakers, those with impaired vision, and those who might require assistance in marking ballots. Studies indicate lower voting rates among persons with disabilities even when a mail-in option is available, but a larger percentage of persons with disabilities take advantage of vote-by-mail compared with the general population.[58] Absentee ballots and vote-by-mail are also not readily available for those who lack a permanent home address or have nonstandard postal addresses, such as Native Americans.[59] Certain populations also could be at a disadvantage when it comes to getting needed information about the absentee process and requirements. There is some evidence that signature matching disproportionately affects younger and minority populations and could lead to higher rates of ballot rejections than for other populations, suggesting

---

[55] National Conference of State Legislatures, "VOPP: Table 10: Who Can Collect and Return an Absentee Ballot Other Than the Voter," webpage, April 21, 2020d.

[56] Heritage Foundation, undated.

[57] Karp and Banducci, 2000; Southwell and Burchett, 2000.

[58] Schur, Ameri, and Adya, 2017.

[59] For an articulation of the challenges that Native Americans face in access, see Native American Rights Fund, "Vote by Mail," webpage, undated. Also see Peter Dunphy, "The State of Native American Voting Rights," Brennan Center for Justice website, March 13, 2019.

that efforts to support integrity could, in some instances, compromise access for some groups of voters.[60] The benefits of absentee voting for access might be greater in a pandemic context if many people wishing to vote are concerned about the safety of doing so in person.

Logistics

Large-scale distribution of absentee ballots, particularly if there is a spike in requests close to a state's deadline, could cause logistical constraints at the front end as election officials work to process requests and send out ballots. Election officials also have to make estimates of how many absentee ballots to print and plan for processing those ballots when they are returned, including verifying whether the voter has properly signed the ballot. Signature verification can be conducted either manually or using signature matching technology (and sometimes a combination of the two). A greater volume of absentee ballots can overwhelm a manual process. Voter errors or other reviews that might lead to rejecting a ballot as illegitimate also might need to address corrective action that the voter has a right to, such as receiving notification of the ballot rejection in time to make corrections where allowed by law.

Processing a larger number of absentee ballots than normally anticipated could require hiring additional workers and procuring equipment, such as high-volume optical scanners. Most ballots will be folded and placed in a privacy sleeve in addition to a mailing envelope. Workers have to extract ballots, sort them, and prepare them for batch scanning. In addition to ballots returned by mail, voting drop-boxes might be needed in accessible places for voters to return their ballots should they choose to do so in this manner. Finally, voters also have to be made aware of the timelines for requesting and returning their ballots.

For states with lower participation rates for either vote-by-mail or absentee voting, transitioning to this option is not a simple task. Oregon's transition to universal vote-by-mail, for example, was a multiyear process that started at the local level in the early 1980s and gradually

---

[60] For example, see the analysis of rejection rates in Florida jurisdictions in Smith, 2018.

evolved into a statewide practice in 2000.[61] States seeking to transition to vote-by-mail, whether universal or on-demand, can learn from the experience of other states, but no state has undertaken converting to vote-by-mail in just a few months. Ensuring that there are certified printers available to handle the greater demand for ballot printing is also an important consideration.[62] Officials also might wish to procure special equipment, such as envelope slicers, to assist in processing (and testing to ensure that they do not accidentally slice ballots).

Equipment purchases—particularly new types of equipment, such as envelope slicers or high-speed optical scanners—are likely to be in high demand and could be back-ordered. Once the new equipment arrives, testing is needed to ensure that workers know how to use the equipment and to identify process bottlenecks or problems that can arise, such as adjusting settings to ensure that ballots are not damaged in processing or misfed. This step in the process includes training for workers regarding high-volume processing, signature verification, chain of custody on ballots, and procedures for ballot errors.

States and jurisdictions that do not have AVR (which can help maintain more-accurate voter registration records) might consider sending a mailer to confirm addresses prior to distributing ballots, given that the expectation is that up to 10 percent of registered voters might have moved without updating their addresses in the system.[63] This added step can improve voter roll accuracy but risks reducing voter responses and removal from registration rolls. Election officials can also check the National Change of Address database in advance of mailing ballots. AVR systems can ease some of these considerations because it improves the ability to maintain up-to-date and accurate voter registration records.

Implementing an automated system or developing a manual process for smaller jurisdictions involves planning out the process flow and physical space for front-end creation of ballot packages prior to mailing and for back-end receipt and processing of completed ballots.

---

[61] Oregon Secretary of State, "Oregon Vote-by-Mail," undated.

[62] U.S. Election Assistance Commission, "Preliminary Planning for Increased Voting by Mail/Absentee Voting," webinar, March 20, 2020.

[63] U.S. Election Assistance Commission, 2020.

Jurisdictions will need to address how to handle large volumes of ballots returned closer to Election Day and the requirements for certifying the election. Certification dates vary by state and sometimes by jurisdiction.[64] For vote-by-mail, many voters wish to return their ballots to a drop-box rather than by mail, particularly if they have to pay for postage. This means that decisions must be made about placing drop-boxes, securing them, and having sufficient workforce to ensure chain of custody from the drop-box to a central processing facility.

Finally, even with automation, many jurisdictions still need to rely on recruiting and hiring temporary workers or volunteers to assist with election processing, including bipartisan teams to address such issues as ballot duplication or analyzing unclear voter intent.

Election officials will need to plan ahead to ensure that an authorized printer can provide an adequate supply of absentee ballots, package those ballots, and distribute them via the postal service. Election officials might wish to hedge against postal delays by distributing ballots earlier than normal. They will also need to plan out the back-end processing and chain of custody, including secure storage of ballots after the election as required by federal law.

The main cost considerations are

- printing and postage costs for additional ballots
- ballot-tracking systems and chain of custody (including storage)
- processing equipment for returned ballots (for example, automated letter openers, sorters, scanners)
- staffing costs.

Summary

Absentee ballots and vote-by-mail provide safe forms of voting given that voters do not need to wait in lines or come into close contact with others in a polling place. Risks associated with health safety are largely eliminated and there could be some increase in access (although there could also be access challenges for specific populations). Risks to integrity remain low but might be higher than for in-

---

[64] U.S. Election Assistance Commission, *Election Management Guidelines: Canvassing and Certifying an Election*, Silver Spring, Md., August 26, 2010.

person options. A primary challenge for election officials, however, is anticipating the volume of ballots needed and ensuring that they are distributed and can be processed in the time frame allowed prior to election certification.

Figure 4.4 presents the states that allow either absentee ballots or vote-by-mail.

Figure 4.4
States by Remote Voting Method

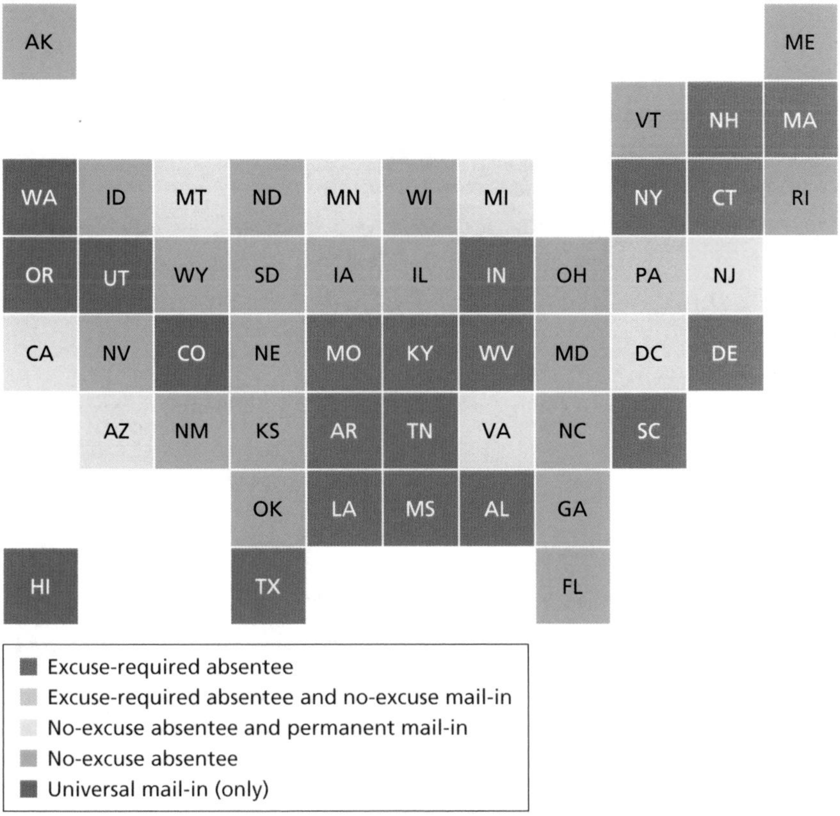
AK
ME
VT
NH
MA
WA
ID
MT
ND
MN
WI
MI
NY
CT
RI
OR
UT
WY
SD
IA
IL
IN
OH
PA
NJ
CA
NV
CO
NE
MO
KY
WV
MD
DC
DE
AZ
NM
KS
AR
TN
VA
NC
SC
OK
LA
MS
AL
GA
HI
TX
FL
Excuse-required absentee
Excuse-required absentee and no-excuse mail-in
No-excuse absentee and permanent mail-in
No-excuse absentee
Universal mail-in (only)

SOURCE: National Conference of State Legislatures, 2020d.

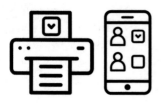

Other Forms of Remote Voting

For completeness, we briefly address other forms of remote voting: voting by fax or electronically through email or a website. These forms of remote voting are attractive from a safety perspective because they limit, and perhaps even eliminate, the need for voters to engage in contact with others except where they might need assistance with access or transmission. Voting by fax is limited in most states to a subset of voters, such as those included under UOCAVA or persons with disabilities. Fax submission of ballots is inherently insecure, however, because they are traditionally sent on unencrypted phone lines.[65]

Online voting is not an option for the broader voting public in any U.S. state. A few states (Delaware, New Jersey, and West Virginia) and localities (for example, the District of Columbia and King County in Washington State) have experimented with forms of web-based or email voting in elections.[66] The cybersecurity concerns over electronic voting are considerable, however, as noted in guidance that the U.S. Department of Homeland Security issued in May 2020 and in recent research on the cybersecurity of electronic voting platforms that enable email or app-based ballot submission.[67] Pilot studies and research on

---

[65] David Jefferson, "What About Email and Fax Voting?" Verified Voting website, undated.

[66] National Conference of State Legislatures, "Electronic Transmission of Ballots," webpage, September 5, 2019b. Also see Miles Parks, "States Expand Internet Voting Experiments Amid Pandemic, Raising Security Fears," National Public Radio, April 28, 2020a; Sophia Schmidt, "Delaware Piloting New Internet-Based Voting System for Disabled, Overseas Voters," Delaware Public Media, May 1, 2020; and Emily S. Rueb, "Voting by Phone Gets a Big Test, but There Are Concerns," *New York Times*, January 23, 2020.

[67] Sean Lyngaas, "DHS Memo: 'Significant' Security Risks Presented by Online Voting," Cyberscoop, May 11, 2020. Also see Sunoo Park, Michael Specter, Neha Nerula, and Ron Rivest, "Going from Bad to Worse: From Internet Voting to Blockchain Voting," draft paper, Massachusetts Institute of Technology, February 20, 2020; Michael A. Specter and J. Alex Halderman, "Security Analysis of the Democracy Live Online Voting System," Internet Policy Research Initiative, white paper, June 7, 2020; and Michael A. Specter, James Koppel, and Daniel Weitzner, "The Ballot is Busted Before the Blockchain: A Security Analysis of Voatz, the First Internet Voting Application Used in U.S. Federal Elections," Internet Policy Research Initiative, white paper, undated.

other countries suggest that online voting can expand access, although the expansion tends to be small. Most who shift to online voting in these studies were inclined to vote anyway.[68] Furthermore, online voting brings new concerns regarding access that are related to the unequal spread of reliable internet and digital technologies.

Summary of Analysis of Factors for Voting Options

Based on the foregoing analysis, we can draw some general conclusions about the risks across the voting options, although the specific considerations will vary by state. Table 4.2 outlines the options available for voting and discusses the relevant considerations along these four dimensions. Again, we do not factor in considerations that apply equally to all options—for example, all options must provide accommodations for non-English speakers and voters with disabilities. Safety risks are high-

Table 4.2
Summary of Risks for Implementing Voting Options During a Pandemic

	Risks to Safety	Risks to Integrity	Risks to Access	Logistical Considerations
In-person (Election Day or early voting)	High (potentially lower with early voting) • New interpersonal contact	Minimal • Possible identification requirement	Moderate • Travel required • Possible identification requirement • Physical requirement	Safety and sanitation mitigations • Communication • Physical space or modifications • Training
Mail (absentee or mail-in)	Minimal	Low (but higher than in-person) • Increased volume of mail-in ballots might increase risk (e.g., harder to detect fraud)	Minimal	Dissemination • Processing and verification • Training • Verification
Other (online or fax)	Minimal	High • Cybersecurity • Technical failures	Low • Internet availability • Technology requirements	Online system, processing • Verification • Training • Communication

---

[68] Solvak and Vassil, 2018; Stromer-Galley, 2003, p. 87.

est for in-person voting, at least in the COVID-19 context. Mitigations are available to help reduce this risk but will involve additional effort and cost. The safety considerations associated with voting on Election Day and voting early are similar; both are in-person processes, although early voting can help spread out voters and reduce the challenges associated with social distancing. Access considerations appear lowest for mail-in voting, although even this approach can create hurdles for some voters, as described earlier. Access concerns are somewhat higher for in-person voting methods (which require people to travel to the polls) and for online voting options (which are restricted, as already described, and which require access to specific technology and to reliable internet connectivity).[69] Early voting also could have some positive effect on increasing access if it offers more flexibility to voters and allows them to vote more easily. However, it is worth noting that research finds only muted effects of early voting on turnout.[70] Integrity concerns are lowest for in-person voting methods and highest for online approaches. Although the risk of fraud is potentially higher for mail-in options than for in-person voting, this risk remains very low, as noted elsewhere. Finally, as was true for registration, there are significant pandemic-related logistical considerations across options. It is hard to compare these options based on scale or to assess which set of logistical considerations is most or least severe. Instead, we assess that, regardless of the options chosen, local officials will need to address a variety of logistical issues, whether these result from physical safety and sanitation issues or from the technical requirements of disseminating, collecting, and processing mail-in ballots.

We can also compare across options, looking specifically at which voting options present the most risks and considerations for local officials within the pandemic context. Table 4.2 would seem to indicate that local officials would need to implement more mitigation for in-person voting than for mail-in voting. Once again, however, this assessment is particular to the current context. Furthermore, the risks and consider-

---

[69] Karp and Banducci, 2000; Solvak and Vassil, 2018; Southwell and Burchett, 2000; Stromer-Galley, 2003, p. 87.

[70] Gronke, Galanes-Rosenbaum, and Miller, 2007; Stein, 1998.

ations across options might have different relevance and different implications in different states. Ultimately, each state must weigh the different considerations outlined here and decide which mix of approaches is best. Some states might lean toward mail-in voting options; others might prefer in-person options. Notably, states will be constrained in their choices by political and legal considerations. In some states, for example, early voting is not permitted by the state constitution.[71] In others, mail-in voting is allowed only with a valid excuse, and the legislative effort to change such a provision might be prohibitive.

---

[71] Kathleen Megan and Jenna Carlesso, "Connecticut Senate Endorses Early Voting but Not with Margin to Get It on 2020 Ballot," *Hartford Courant*, May 8, 2019.

CHAPTER FIVE

Considering a Portfolio of Options for Registration and Voting During a Pandemic

The foregoing analysis of options provides an overview of the factors that election officials, state and local elected officials, and other stakeholders should consider when examining a particular approach to voter registration and vote-casting in the face of a continuing public health emergency. Decisionmakers need to evaluate these options not as mutually exclusive choices but as a set of options that will have to be considered collectively. The options we have laid out in this report provide a view of how each option differs in terms of the ability to provide for worker and voter safety in the COVID-19 context, guard the integrity of elections, promote access for eligible voters, and highlight the logistical considerations (including cost categories).

The first thing to underscore is that no option is entirely free of risk and that the risks in 2020 are not only the same challenges to safety, integrity, and access that always exist but also a whole new set of additional risks and considerations. COVID-19 threatens the health of people who gather and interact; therefore, it poses a direct risk to in-person voters that did not exist previously.

As noted, each state will have to consider the challenges and risks associated with each option and then make decisions about which risks to accept and which to avoid. States are starting from different sets of conditions in terms of election systems that they already have, and states could well find themselves facing different conditions regarding the pandemic come November. Therefore, each state might come to distinct conclusions and offer different options to voters. The purpose of this report is not to tell policymakers or election officials which options to select; rather, it is to lay out the pandemic-related challenges, risks, and other considerations the officials should consider when making their choices.

For example, if a state or jurisdiction decides to transition largely to absentee balloting and reduce in-person voting options, what happens if people feel safe on Election Day and more individuals decide to vote in person than anticipated? This could lead to large crowds and long lines and could make it difficult to maintain social distancing and other health measures while ensuring that everyone can participate in the voting process. If state and local elected officials and election officials choose an option that would require significant voter behavior changes (for example, a state that has low absentee balloting historically but decides to invest in a large number of absentee ballots), there is a risk of mismatching election options with the desires of the voting public—particularly if those changes are not communicated well to that public. Communicating with the voting public is particularly important in the context of potential foreign interference in U.S. elections; such interference might include spreading disinformation on election processes and/or calling their integrity into question. Resources and time are finite, however, and pursuing multiple options can stretch already stressed budgets.[1] In other words, decisionmakers also need ways to bound and quantify uncertainty surrounding COVID-19 and voter behavior, but getting clarity on either will be difficult, especially on the timeline required to be prepared for November.

To assist with determining a risk-informed path forward, we offer a set of filtering questions for state officials to ask themselves.

What is our starting point in terms of election systems and voter preferences? States where most people have historically voted in person are at a different starting point than states where universal vote-by-mail has been implemented, particularly when viewed from a perspective of safety. Similar considerations apply to registration methods.

What types of risks are we willing to accept? What are our risk priorities? States vary in the extent to which they feel that changes to their election processes are required or desirable. Although all states might choose to implement some health-related precautions at in-person voting locations, some states might lean toward efforts to expand mail-in voting while others might prefer to continue with existing processes augmented by additional polling locations or expanded early voting. Although many factors will be considered, at least part of the decision will be based on the preferences and risk tolerance of key stakeholders.

How much flexibility is there to make changes to our existing approach? States also have different laws and regulations around voting and so vary in the ease with which they can modify policy and practice on the timeline required. States and jurisdictions that have less flexibility, such as those that require legislative changes to allow for no-excuse absentee ballots or vote-by-mail, could have fewer choices in the near term when it comes to changing voting methods and might instead choose to focus more closely on implementing safety precautions and communicating those measures broadly to the voting public.[2]

Given estimates of uncertainty and voter preferences, do we have the capacity to meet voter demands for different types of voting options? Historical experience and estimates of 2020 turnout and voter preferences (which could be gleaned from new or existing studies) indicate that state officials should be able to produce rough estimates of how many eligible voters might turn out to vote in person on Election Day, vote early, or take advantage of mail-in options (where those exist). Such estimates could allow state officials to determine whether existing capacity is sufficient for in-person, mail-in, and other options—and if it is not, what additional mix of policy options might be required to meet demand (for example, more in-person locations or additional in-person mitigations and some additional remote voting) and what additional costs (both monetary and potentially political) these modifications might entail. Finally, it is worth noting that to truly hedge against uncertainty, planners might choose to slightly overestimate demand across methods or develop the capacity to rapidly shift staff or resources from one voting method to another as late as Election Day; if they do so, these changes should be broadly communicated to the voting public.

Elected officials, policymakers, and election officials face extraordinary circumstances preparing for the November election. Planning under such uncertain conditions will require careful evaluation and likely additional funding from states—and the federal government, given the strain on state and local budgets stemming from the response to the COVID-19 pandemic.

References

Armitage, Susie, "Mail-In Ballot Postage Becomes a Surprising (and Unnecessary) Cause of Voter Anxiety," *ProPublica*, November 1, 2018. As of June 23, 2020: https://www.propublica.org/article/mail-in-ballot-postage-becomes-a-surprising-and-unnecessary-cause-of-voter-anxiety

Associated Press, "Voter Registrations Slow with Virus Closing DMV Offices," *US News and World Report*, April 2, 2020. As of May 28, 2020: https://www.usnews.com/news/best-states/nevada/articles/2020-04-02/voter-registrations-slow-with-virus-closing-dmv-offices

Barreto, Matt A., Mara Cohen-Marks, and Nathan D. Woods, "Are All Precincts Created Equal? The Prevalence of Low-Quality Precincts in Low-Income and Minority Communities," *Political Research Quarterly*, Vol. 62, No. 3, September 2009, pp. 445–458.

Barreto, Matt, Chad Dunn, Vivian Alejandre, Michael Cohen, Tye Rush, and Sonni Waknin, *Protecting Democracy: Implementing Equal and Safe Access to the Ballot Box During a Global Pandemic*, Los Angeles, Calif.: UCLA Latino Policy and Politics Initiative, March 23, 2020.

Brito, Christopher, "CDC Director Says Potentially Worse Second Wave of Coronavirus Could Come Along with Flu Season," CBS News, April 23, 2020. As of May 25, 2020: https://www.cbsnews.com/news/coronavirus-second-wave-cdc-director-robert-redfield-warning-flu-season/

Center for Civic Design, *Design Documentation: Vote-by-Mail Envelope Design for California*, Omaha, Neb.: Oxide Design Co, December 15, 2017. As of June 27, 2020: https://elections.cdn.sos.ca.gov/vote-by-mail/pdf/guidance.pdf

Centers for Disease Control and Prevention, "How to Protect Yourself & Others," webpage, April 24, 2020a. As of May 28, 2020: https://www.cdc.gov/coronavirus/2019-ncov/prevent-getting-sick/prevention.html

Centers for Disease Control and Prevention, "Older Adults," webpage, April 30, 2020b. As of June 8, 2020:
https://www.cdc.gov/coronavirus/2019-ncov/need-extra-precautions/older-adults.html

Centers for Disease Control and Prevention, "Social Distancing," webpage, May 6, 2020c. As of June 8, 2020:
https://www.cdc.gov/coronavirus/2019-ncov/prevent-getting-sick/social-distancing.html

Commission on Federal Election Reform, *Building Confidence in U.S. Elections: Report of The Commission on Federal Election Reform*, September 2005. As of July 14, 2020:
https://www.legislationline.org/download/id/1472/file/3b50795b2d0374cbef5c29766256.pdf

Cook County Clerk's Office, "Register to Vote," webpage, undated. As of June 20, 2020:
https://www.cookcountyclerk.com/agency/register-vote

Corasaniti, Nick, and Stephanie Saul, "Requests for Vote-by-Mail Ballot Overwhelm the Elections Agency in New York City," *New York Times*, June 20, 2020.

Cortina, Jeronimo, and Brandon Rottinghaus, "'The Quiet Revolution': Convenience Voting, Vote Centers, and Turnout in Texas Elections," conference paper presented to the Election Sciences, Reform, and Administration Conference, University of Pennsylvania, 2019. As of June 7, 2020:
https://cpb-us-w2.wpmucdn.com/web.sas.upenn.edu/dist/7/538/files/2019/06/Cortina-and-Rottinghaus-ESRA-2019-Paper.pdf

"Court Says Kansas Can't Require Voters to Show Citizenship Proof," PBS Newshour website, April 29, 2020. As of June 19, 2020:
https://www.pbs.org/newshour/politics/court-says-kansas-cant-require-voters-to-show-citizenship-proof

Cybersecurity and Infrastructure Security Agency, "#Protect2020," webpage, June 3, 2020. As of June 10, 2020:
https://www.cisa.gov/protect2020

Deluzio, Christopher R., Elizabeth Howard, David Levine, Paul Rosenzweig, and Derek Tisler, *Ensuring Safe Elections: Federal Funding Needs for State and Local Governments During the Pandemic*, New York: Brennan Center for Justice, April 30, 2020.

Dirr, Alison, and Mary Spicuzza, "What We Know So Far About Why Milwaukee Only Had 5 Voting Sites for Tuesday's Election While Madison Had 66," *Milwaukee Journal Sentinel*, April 9, 2020. As of June 2, 2020:
https://www.jsonline.com/story/news/politics/elections/2020/04/09/wisconsin-election-milwaukee-had-5-voting-sites-while-madison-had-66/2970587001/

van Doremale, Neeltje, Trenton Bushmaker, Dylan H. Morris, Myndi G. Holbrook, Amandine Gamble, Brandi Williamson, Azaibi Tamin, Jennifer L. Harcourt, Natalie J. Thornburg, Susan I. Gerber, James O. Lloyd-Smith, Emmei de Wit, and Vincent Munster, "Aerosol and Surface Stability of SARS-CoV-2 as Compared with SARS-CoV-1," *New England Journal of Medicine*, Vol. 382, No. 16, March 2020.

Dunphy, Peter, "The State of Native American Voting Rights," Brennan Center for Justice website, March 13, 2019. As of June 2, 2020:
https://www.brennancenter.org/our-work/analysis-opinion/state-native-american-voting-rights

Electronic Registration Information Center, homepage, undated. As of June 10, 2020:
https://ericstates.org

Fausset, Richard, Reid J. Epstein, and Rick Rojas, "Anger and Mistrust in Georgia as Vote Dissolves into Debacle," *New York Times*, June 10, 2020.

Federal Voting Assistance Program, "Election Forms and Tools for Sending," webpage, undated-a. As of May 25, 2020:
https://www.fvap.gov/eo/overview/materials/forms

Federal Voting Assistance Program, homepage, undated-b. As of June 20, 2020:
https://www.fvap.gov

Federal Voting Assistance Program, "Voter Registration and Ballots," webpages for military and overseas citizens, undated-c. As of June 20, 2020:
https://www.fvap.gov/military-voter/registration-ballots
https://www.fvap.gov/citizen-voter/registration-ballots

Franklin, Daniel P., and Eric E. Grier, "Effects of Motor Voter Legislation: Voter Turnout, Registration, and Partisan Advantage in the 1992 Presidential Election," *American Politics Quarterly*, Vol. 25, No. 1, 1997, pp. 104–117.

Garisto, Daniel, "Smartphone Data Show Voters in Black Neighborhoods Wait Longer," *Scientific American*, October 1, 2019. As of June 9, 2020:
https://www.scientificamerican.com/article/smartphone-data-show-voters-in-black-neighborhoods-wait-longer1/

Goel, Sharad, Marc Meredith, Michael Morse, David Rothschild, and Houshmand Shirani-Mehr, "One Person, One Vote: Estimating the Prevalence of Double Voting in U.S. Presidential Elections," *American Political Science Review*, Vol. 114, No. 2, May 2020, pp. 456–469.

Gronke, Paul, Eva Galanes-Rosenbaum, and Peter A. Miller, "Early Voting and Turnout," *PS: Political Science & Politics*, Vol. 40, No. 4, 2007, pp. 639–645.

Hajnal, Zoltan, Nazita Lajevardi, and Lindsay Nielson, "Voter Identification Laws and the Suppression of Minority Votes," *Journal of Politics*, Vol. 79, No. 2, 2017, pp. 363–379.

Harvard Medical School, "Coronavirus Outbreak and Kids," June 11, 2020. As of June 21, 2020:
https://www.health.harvard.edu/diseases-and-conditions/coronavirus-outbreak-and-kids

Heritage Foundation, "A Sampling of Recent Election Fraud Cases from Across the United States," database, undated. As of June 20, 2020:
https://www.heritage.org/voterfraud

Highton, Benjamin, "Voter Identification Laws and Turnout in the United States," *Annual Review of Political Science*, Vol. 20, 2017, pp. 149–167.

Institute for Health Metrics and Evaluation, "COVID-19 Projections," webpage, July 14, 2020. As of July 15, 2020:
https://covid19.healthdata.org/united-states-of-america

Jefferson, David, "What About Email and Fax Voting?" Verified Voting website, undated. As of June 2, 2020:
https://www.verifiedvoting.org/resources/internet-voting/email-fax/

Karp, Jeffrey A., and Susan A. Banducci, "Going Postal: How All-Mail Elections Influence Turnout," *Political Behavior*, Vol. 22, No. 3, 2000, pp. 223–239.

Kavanagh, Jennifer, Quentin E. Hodgson, C. Ben Gibson, and Samantha Cherney, *An Assessment of State Voting Processes: Preparing for Elections During a Pandemic*, Santa Monica, Calif.: RAND Corporation, RR-A112-8, 2020. As of August 2020:
https://www.rand.org/pubs/research_reports/RRA112-8.html

Kavanagh, Jennifer, and Michael D. Rich, *Truth Decay: An Initial Exploration of the Diminishing Role of Facts and Analysis in American Public Life*, Santa Monica, Calif.: RAND Corporation, RR-2314-RC, 2018. As of July 13, 2020:
https://www.rand.org/pubs/research_reports/RR2314.html

Kissler, Stephen M., Christine Tedijanto, Edward Goldstein, Yonatan H. Grad, and Marc Lipsitch, "Projecting the Transmission Dynamics of SARS-CoV-2 Through the Postpandemic Period," *Science*, Vol. 368, No. 6493, 2020, pp. 860–868.

Klain, Hannah, Kevin Morris, Max Feldman, and Rebecca Ayala, *Waiting to Vote: Racial Disparities in Election Day Experiences*, New York: Brennan Center for Justice, June 3, 2020. As of June 21, 2020:
https://www.brennancenter.org/sites/default/files/2020-06/6_02_WaitingtoVote_FINAL.pdf

Klobuchar, Amy, "Amy Klobuchar: The Right Way to Vote This November," *New York Times*, April 14, 2020.

Knack, Stephen, "Does 'Motor Voter' Work? Evidence from State-Level Data," *Journal of Politics*, Vol. 57, No. 3, 1995, pp. 796–811.

Korecki, Natasha, and Zach Montellaro, "Wisconsin Supreme Court Overturns Governor, Orders Tuesday Elections to Proceed," *Politico*, April 6, 2020. As of April 23, 2020:
https://www.politico.com/news/2020/04/06/
wisconsin-governor-orders-stop-to-in-person-voting-on-eve-of-election-168527

Logan, Mia, "These States Allow Online Voting for Citizens, Is Your State One of Them?" *eBallot* blog, May 16, 2019. As of May 25, 2020:
https://www.eballot.com/blog/
these-states-allow-online-voting-for-their-citizens-is-your-state-one-of-them

Lyngaas, Sean, "DHS Memo: 'Significant' Security Risks Presented by Online Voting," Cyberscoop, May 11, 2020. As of June 1, 2020:
https://www.cyberscoop.com/dhs-cisa-online-voting-risks/

Matsubayashi, Tetsuya, and Michiko Ueda, "Disability and Voting," *Disability and Health Journal*, Vol. 7, 2014, pp. 285–291.

McGhee, Eric, and Mindy Romero, *Effects of Automatic Voter Registration in the United States*, Los Angeles, Calif.: USC Sol Price School of Public Policy, 2020.

Megan, Kathleen, and Jenna Carlesso, "Connecticut Senate Endorses Early Voting but Not with Margin to Get It on 2020 Ballot," *Hartford Courant*, May 8, 2019.

Minnite, Lori, and David Callahan, *Securing the Vote*, New York: Demos, 2003.

Missouri Secretary of State, "How to Vote," webpage, undated. As of June 10, 2020:
https://www.sos.mo.gov/elections/goVoteMissouri/howtovote

Moore, Kristine A., Marc Lipsitch, John M. Barry, and Michael T. Osterholm, *COVID-19: The CIDRAP Viewpoint*, Part 1, *The Future of the COVID-19 Pandemic: Lessons Learned from Pandemic Influenza*, Minneapolis, Minn.: Center for Infectious Disease Research and Policy, University of Minnesota, April 30, 2020. As of May 25, 2020:
https://www.cidrap.umn.edu/sites/default/files/public/downloads/
cidrap-covid19-viewpoint-part1_0.pdf

Morley, Michael T., and Franita Tolson, "Elections Clause," *Interactive Constitution* website, undated. As of May 25, 2020:
https://constitutioncenter.org/interactive-constitution/interpretation/article-i/
clauses/750

Morris, Kevin, and Peter Dunphy, *AVR Impact on State Voter Registration*, New York: Brennan Center for Justice, 2019. As of June 23, 2020:
https://www.brennancenter.org/sites/default/files/2019-08/Report_AVR_Impact_
State_Voter_Registration.pdf

Mycoff, Jason D., Michael W. Wagner, and David C. Wilson, "The Empirical Effects of Voter-ID Laws: Present or Absent?" *Political Science and Politics*, Vol. 41, No. 1, January 2009, pp. 121–126.

National Conference of State Legislatures, "Voter Verification Without ID Documents," webpage, undated. As of June 21, 2020:
https://www.ncsl.org/research/elections-and-campaigns/
voter-verification-without-id-documents.aspx

National Conference of State Legislatures, "Legislative Session Length," webpage, December 2, 2010. As of June 10, 2020:
https://www.ncsl.org/research/about-state-legislatures/legislative-session-length.aspx

National Conference of State Legislatures, "Voter Registration," webpage, September 27, 2016. As of May 25, 2020:
https://www.ncsl.org/research/elections-and-campaigns/voter-registration.aspx

National Conference of State Legislatures, "Access to and Use of Voter Registration Lists," webpage, August 5, 2019a. As of June 21, 2020:
https://www.ncsl.org/research/elections-and-campaigns/
access-to-and-use-of-voter-registration-lists.aspx

National Conference of State Legislatures, "Electronic Transmission of Ballots," webpage, September 5, 2019b. As of June 2, 2020:
https://www.ncsl.org/research/elections-and-campaigns/internet-voting.aspx

National Conference of State Legislatures, "Verification of Absentee Ballots," webpage, January 21, 2020a. As of June 14, 2020:
https://www.ncsl.org/research/elections-and-campaigns/
verification-of-absentee-ballots.aspx

National Conference of State Legislatures, "Online Voter Registration," webpage, February 3, 2020b. As of June 4, 2020:
https://www.ncsl.org/research/elections-and-campaigns/
electronic-or-online-voter-registration.aspx

National Conference of State Legislatures, "Voter List Accuracy," webpage, March 20, 2020c. As of May 25, 2020:
https://www.ncsl.org/research/elections-and-campaigns/voter-list-accuracy.aspx

National Conference of State Legislatures, "VOPP: Table 10: Who Can Collect and Return an Absentee Ballot Other Than the Voter," webpage, April 21, 2020d. As of June 21, 2020:
https://www.ncsl.org/research/elections-and-campaigns/vopp-table-10-who-can-collect-and-return-an-absentee-ballot-other-than-the-voter.aspx

Native American Rights Fund, "Vote by Mail," webpage, undated. As of June 8, 2020:
https://www.narf.org/vote-by-mail/

New Jersey Division of Elections, "Register to Vote!" webpage, June 16, 2020. As of June 20, 2020:
https://www.state.nj.us/state/elections/voter-registration.shtml

Newman, Lily Hay, "Vote by Mail Isn't Perfect. But It's Essential in a Pandemic," *Wired*, April 9, 2020. As of May 25, 2020:
https://www.wired.com/story/
vote-by-mail-absentee-coronvirus-covid-19-pandemic/

Norden, Lawrence, Aaron Burstein, Joseph Lorenzo Hall, and Margaret Chen, *Post-Election Audits: Restoring Trust in Elections: Executive Summary*, New York: Brennan Center for Justice and Samuelson Law, Technology & Public Policy Clinic, 2007.

Oklahoma State Election Board, "Online Voter Registration," webpage, November 1, 2019. As of May 7, 2020:
https://www.ok.gov/elections/Online_Voter_Registration.html

Oregon Secretary of State, "Oregon Vote-by-Mail," webpage, undated. As of June 2, 2020:
https://sos.oregon.gov/elections/Documents/statistics/vote-by-mail-timeline.pdf

Park, Sunoo, Michael Specter, Neha Nerula, and Ron Rivest, "Going from Bad to Worse: From Internet Voting to Blockchain Voting," draft paper, Massachusetts Institute of Technology, February 20, 2020.

Parker-Pope, Tara, "What's the Risk of Catching Coronavirus from a Surface?" *New York Times*, June 3, 2020.

Parks, Miles, "States Expand Internet Voting Experiments Amid Pandemic, Raising Security Fears," National Public Radio, April 28, 2020a. As of June 4, 2020:
https://www.npr.org/2020/04/28/844581667/
states-expand-internet-voting-experiments-amid-pandemic-raising-security-fears

Parks, Miles, "Feds Warn States That Online Voting Experiments Are 'High-Risk,'" National Public Radio, May 11, 2020b. As of June 5, 2020:
https://www.npr.org/2020/05/11/853759878/
feds-warn-states-that-online-voting-experiments-are-high-risk

Pazniokas, Mark, and Ana Radelat, "On Easing Absentee Voting, Connecticut Looks to November and Beyond," *CT Mirror*, May 23, 2020. As of June 1, 2020:
https://ctmirror.org/2020/05/23/
on-easing-absentee-voting-connecticut-looks-to-november-and-beyond/

Pew Charitable Trusts, "Online Voter Registration: Trends in Development and Implementation," May 2015. As of June 8, 2020:
https://www.pewtrusts.org/-/media/assets/2015/05/ovr_2015_brief.pdf

Pew Research Center, "An Examination of the 2016 Electorate, Based on Validated Voters," webpage, August 9, 2018. As of June 22, 2020:
https://www.people-press.org/2018/08/09/
an-examination-of-the-2016-electorate-based-on-validated-voters/

Phillips, Amber, "Examining the Arguments Against Voting by Mail," *Washington Post*, May 20, 2020.

Rakich, Nathaniel, "Few States Are Prepared to Switch to Voting by Mail. That Could Make for a Messy Election," *FiveThirtyEight*, April 27, 2020. As of June 8, 2020:
https://fivethirtyeight.com/features/few-states-are-prepared-to-switch-to-voting-by-mail-that-could-make-for-a-messy-election/

Reality Check Team, "US Election: Do Postal Ballots Lead to Voting Fraud?" BBC, July 15, 2020. As of July 16, 2020:
https://www.bbc.com/news/world-us-canada-53353404

Rouan, Rick, "Here's What You Need to Know About Ohio's Delayed Primary Election," *Columbus Dispatch*, April 26, 2020. As of June 7, 2020:
https://www.dispatch.com/news/20200426/
herersquos-what-you-need-to-know-about-ohiorsquos-delayed-primary-election

Rueb, Emily S., "Voting by Phone Gets a Big Test, but There Are Concerns," *New York Times*, January 23, 2020.

Schmidt, Sophia, "Delaware Piloting New Internet-Based Voting System for Disabled, Overseas Voters," Delaware Public Media, May 1, 2020. As of June 8, 2020:
https://www.delawarepublic.org/post/
delaware-piloting-new-internet-based-voting-system-disabled-overseas-voters

Schur, Lisa, Mason Ameri, and Meera Adya, "Disability, Voter Turnout, and Polling Place Accessibility," *Social Science Quarterly*, Vol. 98, No. 5, November 2017, pp. 1374–1390.

Smith, Daniel A., "Vote-by-Mail Ballots Cast in Florida," ACLU Florida webpage, September 19, 2018. As of June 20, 2020:
https://www.aclufl.org/en/publications/vote-mail-ballots-cast-florida

Snead, Jason, *The Unnecessary Risks of Mandated and Rushed Vote-by-Mail*, Honest Elections Project, July 2020. As of July 14, 2020:
https://www.honestelections.org/wp-content/uploads/2020/07/VoteByMail.pdf

Solvak, Mihkel, and Kristjan Vassil, "Could Internet Voting Halt Declining Electoral Turnout? New Evidence That E-Voting Is Habit-Forming," *Policy & Internet*, Vol. 10, No. 1, 2018, pp. 4–21.

Southwell, Priscilla, "In the Pandemic, Every State Should Vote by Mail," *The Atlantic*, April 14, 2020. As of May 25, 2020:
https://www.theatlantic.com/ideas/archive/2020/04/
moral-urgency-voting-mail/609928/

Southwell, Priscilla L., and Justin I. Burchett, "The Effect of All-Mail Elections on Voter Turnout," *American Politics Quarterly*, Vol. 28, No. 1, 2000, pp. 72–79.

Specter, Michael A., and J. Alex Halderman, "Security Analysis of the Democracy Live Online Voting System," Internet Policy Research Initiative, white paper, June 7, 2020. As of June 10, 2020:
https://internetpolicy.mit.edu/wp-content/uploads/2020/06/OmniBallot.pdf

Specter, Michael A., James Koppel, and Daniel Weitzner, "The Ballot is Busted Before the Blockchain: A Security Analysis of Voatz, the First Internet Voting Application Used in U.S. Federal Elections," Internet Policy Research Initiative, white paper, undated. As of June 10, 2020:
https://internetpolicy.mit.edu/wp-content/uploads/2020/02/
SecurityAnalysisOfVoatz_Public.pdf

Starks, Tim, "Snapshots of How the Pandemic Is Influencing Election Security," *Politico Morning Cybersecurity*, June 8, 2020. As of June 8, 2020:
https://www.politico.com/newsletters/morning-cybersecurity/2020/06/08/
snapshots-of-how-the-pandemic-is-influencing-election-security-788331

State of Mississippi, "Mississippi Mail-In Voter Registration Application," online form, undated. As of June 20, 2020:
http://www.msvoterid.ms.gov/forms/Voter_Registration.pdf

State of Utah, "Information for Voters with Disabilities," webpage, undated. As of May 25, 2020:
https://voteinfo.utah.gov/information-for-voters-with-disabilities/

Stein, Robert M., "Introduction: Early Voting," *Public Opinion Quarterly*, Vol. 62, No. 1, 1998, pp. 57–69.

Stein, Robert M., *The Incidence and Detection of Ineligible Voting*, paper presented at American Political Science Association 2013 annual meeting, 2013.

Steinhauser, Paul, "Michigan Says All Voters Will Be Sent Absentee Ballot Applications," Fox News, May 19, 2020. As of June 1, 2020:
https://www.foxnews.com/politics/
michigan-says-that-all-voters-will-be-sent-absentee-ballot-applications

Stewart, Charles, III, Stephen Ansolabehere, and Nathaniel Persily, "Revisiting Public Opinion on Voter Identification and Voter Fraud in an Era of Increasing Partisan Polarization," *Stanford Law Review*, Vol. 68, 2016.

Stromer-Galley, Jennifer, "Will Internet Voting Increase Turnout?" in Philip N. Howard and Steve Jones, eds., *Society Online: The Internet in Context*, Washington, D.C.: SAGE Publications, 2003, Chapter Six.

Sun, Lena H., "CDC Director Warns Second Wave of Coronavirus Is Likely to Be Even More Devastating," *Washington Post*, April 21, 2020.

Underhill, Wendy, "Voter Identification Requirements: Voter ID Laws," National Conference of State Legislatures webpage, February 24, 2020, Table 2. As of June 7, 2020:
https://www.ncsl.org/research/elections-and-campaigns/voter-id.aspx

U.S. Code, Title 3, The President, Chapter 1, Presidential Elections and Vacancies, Section 1, Time of Appointing Electors. As of June 10, 2020:
https://www.law.cornell.edu/uscode/text/3/1

U.S. Code, Title 52, Voting and Elections, Subtitle II, Voting Assistance and Election Administration, Chapter 201, Voting Accessibility for the Elderly and Handicapped. As of June 20, 2020:
https://www.law.cornell.edu/uscode/text/52/subtitle-II/chapter-201

U.S. Department of Justice, "A Guide to Disability Rights Laws," webpage, February 2020a. As of June 10, 2020:
https://www.ada.gov/cguide.htm#anchor62335

U.S. Department of Justice, "Statutes Enforced by the Voting Section," webpage, March 11, 2020b. As of June 21, 2020:
https://www.justice.gov/crt/statutes-enforced-voting-section

U.S. Election Assistance Commission, "National Mail Voter Registration Form," webpage, undated-a. As of June 15, 2020:
https://www.eac.gov/voters/national-mail-voter-registration-form

U.S. Election Assistance Commission, "Vendor and Manufacturer Guidance on Cleaning Voting Machines and Other Election Technology," webpage, undated-b. As of June 10, 2020:
https://www.eac.gov/election-officials/
vendor-and-manufacturer-guidance-cleaning-voting-machines-and-other-election

U.S. Election Assistance Commission, *Election Management Guidelines: Canvassing and Certifying an Election*, Silver Spring, Md., August 26, 2010, pp. 133–138. As of June 8, 2020:
https://www.eac.gov/sites/default/files/eac_assets/1/6/EMG_chapt_13_august_26_2010.pdf

U.S. Election Assistance Commission, "Preliminary Planning for Increased Voting by Mail/Absentee Voting," webinar, March 20, 2020. As of June 2, 2020:
https://www.eac.gov/election-officials/voting-by-mail-absentee-voting

U.S. Postal Service, "Election Mail," webpage, undated. As of June 26, 2020:
https://about.usps.com/gov-services/election-mail/

Vasilogambros, Matt, "Few People Want to Be Poll Workers, and That's a Problem," *Stateline*, October 22, 2018. As of June 8, 2020:
https://www.pewtrusts.org/en/research-and-analysis/blogs/stateline/2018/10/22/
few-people-want-to-be-poll-workers-and-thats-a-problem

Vasilogambros, Matt, "Glitches in California Embolden Automatic Voter Registration Foes," *Stateline*, October 17, 2019. As of June 23, 2020:
https://www.pewtrusts.org/en/research-and-analysis/blogs/stateline/2019/10/17/
glitches-in-california-embolden-automatic-voter-registration-foes

Verified Voting, "The Verifier—Polling Place Equipment—November 2020," webpage, undated. As of June 8, 2020:
https://www.verifiedvoting.org/verifier/

Viesbeck, Elise, "Tiny Rate of Fraudulent Ballots Undercuts Claims of Risk," *Washington Post*, June 9, 2020.

VoteRiders, "What's the Difference Between Voter ID and Voter Registration?" webpage, undated. As of June 10, 2020:
https://www.voteriders.org/ufaqs/difference-voter-id-voter-registration/

Washington State, "Elections," webpage, undated. As of June 20, 2020:
https://www.sos.wa.gov/elections/print-voter-registration-forms.aspx

Zetter, Kim, "U.S. Government Plans to Urge States to Resist 'High-Risk' Internet Voting," *The Guardian*, May 8, 2020. As of July 6, 2020:
https://www.theguardian.com/us-news/2020/may/08/
us-government-internet-voting-department-of-homeland-security

About the Authors

Quentin E. Hodgson is a senior international and defense researcher at the RAND Corporation focusing on cybersecurity, cyber operations, critical infrastructure protection, risk management, and command and control. He has led projects for the U.S. Department of Defense, the U.S. Department of Homeland Security, and NATO's Allied Command Transformation. He holds an M.A. in international relations and an M.Sc. in national resource management, and was a Fulbright scholar affiliated with the University of Potsdam, Germany.

Jennifer Kavanagh is a senior political scientist at the RAND Corporation and director of the Strategy, Doctrine, and Resources Program in the RAND Arroyo Center. She also leads RAND's Countering Truth Decay initiative, a portfolio of projects exploring the diminishing reliance on facts and analysis in U.S. political and civil discourse. Her research focuses on U.S. defense strategy, international conflict, disinformation, and the relationship between U.S. political and media institutions. She earned her Ph.D. in political science and public policy.

Anusree Garg is a policy analyst at the RAND Corporation. She earned her J.D. in international law.

Edward W. Chan is a senior operations researcher at the RAND Corporation with a background in mathematical modeling, simulation, and optimization. His research has covered a diverse array of applications, including homeland security, logistics, health, and emergency preparedness. He earned his Ph.D. in operations research.

Christine Sovak is a user experience designer at the RAND Corporation She has an M.S. in media arts and technology and is UX Certified through the Nielsen Norman Group, with advanced specializations in UX Management and Interaction Design.